Schizophrenia

Schizophrenia: A Contemporary Introduction provides a vital overview of psychoanalytic work with patients dealing with schizophrenia, highlighting the many benefits of this approach and introducing key methods for mental health practitioners.

This concise introductory volume starts by offering a brief historical introduction to how psychoanalysts, from Freud onwards, have approached schizophrenia and the methods they have used to alleviate the distress it causes its sufferers. Gillian Steggles illustrates how the developing relationship between patient and analyst can positively impact the patient's mental functioning, leading to an improvement in their overall health and the ability to regain independence and self-reliance. She introduces theoretical psychoanalytic approaches, such as the Psychodynamic Pentapointed Cognitive Construct (PPCC) model, as a means of offering guidance to analysts dealing with schizophrenic analysands.

This book will be of interest to practicing and trainee analysts, as well as those interested in the history of schizophrenia and its continued impact.

Gillian Steggles is an academic psychiatry researcher based in London. She has a degree in Medicine from University College Hospital, London, and a PhD in Psychoanalytic Studies from Essex University, and her work centres on a psychoanalytic and psychotherapeutic approach to schizophrenia.

Routledge Introductions to Contemporary Psychoanalysis
Aner Govrin, *Ph.D.*
Series Editor
Yael Peri Herzovich, *Ph.D.*
Executive Editor
Itamar Ezer
Assistant Editor

"Routledge Introductions to Contemporary Psychoanalysis" is one of the prominent psychoanalytic publishing ventures of our day. It will comprise dozens of books that will serve as concise introductions dedicated to influential concepts, theories, leading figures, and techniques in psychoanalysis covering every important aspect of psychoanalysis.

The length of each book is fixed at 40,000 words.

The series' books are designed to be easily accessible to provide informative answers in various areas of psychoanalytic thought. Each book will provide updated ideas on topics relevant to contemporary psychoanalysis – from the unconscious and dreams, projective identification and eating disorders, through neuropsychoanalysis, colonialism, and spiritual-sensitive psychoanalysis. Books will also be dedicated to prominent figures in the field, such as Melanie Klein, Jaque Lacan, Sandor Ferenczi, Otto Kernberg, and Michael Eigen.

Not serving solely as an introduction for beginners, the purpose of the series is to offer compendiums of information on particular topics within different psychoanalytic schools. We ask authors to review a topic but also address the readers with their own personal views and contribution to the specific chosen field. Books will make intricate ideas comprehensible without compromising their complexity.

We aim to make contemporary psychoanalysis more accessible to both clinicians and the general educated public.

Transgenerational Trauma: A Contemporary Introduction
Jill Salberg and Sue Grand

Schizophrenia: A Contemporary Introduction
Gillian Steggles

For more information about this series, please visit: www.routledge.com/Routledge-Introductions-to-Contemporary-Psychoanalysis/book-series

Schizophrenia

A Contemporary Introduction

Gillian Steggles

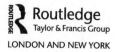
Routledge
Taylor & Francis Group

LONDON AND NEW YORK

Designed cover image: Michal Heiman, Asylum 1855-2020, The Sleeper (video, psychoanalytic sofa and Plate 34), exhibition view, Herzliya Museum of Contemporary Art, 2017

First published 2024
by Routledge
4 Park Square, Milton Park, Abingdon, Oxon OX14 4RN

and by Routledge
605 Third Avenue, New York, NY 10158

Routledge is an imprint of the Taylor & Francis Group, an informa business

British Library Cataloguing-in-Publication Data
A catalogue record for this book is available from the British Library

ISBN: 9781032560397 (hbk)
ISBN: 9781032560380 (pbk)
ISBN: 9781003433507 (ebk)

DOI: 10.4324/9781003433507

Typeset in Times New Roman
by codeMantra

Dedicated to the Psychiatric and Psychoanalytic professions, and wishing them well in their joint endeavours of Psychiatric Psychoanalytic psychotherapy for patients with schizophrenic illness.

Contents

Figures & Table

Figures

Table

A brief foreword

Bob Hinshelwood
Professor R D Hinshelwood

Professor R D Hinshelwood is a Fellow of the British Psychoanalytic Society, a Fellow of the Royal College of Psychiatrists, and Professor Emeritus, University of Essex, UK. He has written widely on psychoanalysis as well as its application to psychiatry and to the dynamics of organisations.

This deeply committed account of distressed patients labelled schizophrenic is sympathetic and insightful into the ways such people experience themselves, others, and their own lives. Despite the usual alienation, this book convincingly presents us with the fact that schizophrenia is not just an illness without there being a person who suffers from it.

It is all too easy in the medical setting, where people so often reside and may even be incarcerated, to picture a set of physiological mechanisms gone wrong. But, walking beside everyone with these symptoms is an essentially human person. Again and again, we are introduced to the fact that we must meet the person. The emphasis is on the meanings their experiences have, meanings that may be confused by them, or conflicted and therefore they avoid them. The caring staff, too, are invariably confused, conflicted, and often avoidant in consequence.

We are accustomed to the increasing importance of a medical suppression of symptoms. But, this book reminds us that, as we treat the symptoms seen from outside, there is also an inside that yearns to be understood and desires to convey that lonely terror by evoking it. Being with those subjective meanings is an essential therapeutic stance just as much as medication intervenes at the level of the brain. Both need to be in balance, but with a slow trend towards meanings more than medications.

This book presents the reader, the patient's family, friends, and acquaintances with the stunning sense of alienation whilst inviting a view through a deeper tunnel into a world of confusion meaninglessness and fear. So, there is a real challenge in introducing the non-professional reader to severe mental disorders since by their very nature such people are excluded from ordinary family and communities. But the challenge is well met by the author. The message is presented with persistence and conviction. No one is just a list of symptoms, and no one is just an illness. Anyone acquainted with people who suffer psychotic states, whether friend, family, acquaintance, or professional, should read this and reflect on the human condition, in general.

Acknowledgements

Grateful thanks are extended to University College London and University College Hospital, London; to the Psychoanalysis Unit at UCL; to the Institute of Psychiatry, Psychology and Neuroscience and to the Maudsley Hospital, in South London; to the Centre for Psychoanalytic Studies at Essex University; to Dr Michael Robbins and to Dr Alec R Tandy; to Professor John Hinton, Dr Murray Jackson, Dr Leslie Sohn, Professor R D Hinshelwood, Professor Julian Leff, Professor Peter Fonagy, Dr Tim Billington, Dr Tim Scannell, Dr Anthony Kaiser, and Dr David MacSweeney; and to the Psychiatry and Psychoanalysis professions for their inspiration and expertise; and infinitely to Mr Trevitt Steggles.

Introduction

A historical review

From the days of the Enlightenment in the 18th century, and even in previous eras, doctors and social reformers have tried to tend and ameliorate incapacitating human distress and madness. Psychiatrists then tried to distinguish, from this, recognisable and salient patterns of illness that they could classify and use to develop treatments. They strove to treat the ravages of illness they could identify with remedies as diverse as straitjackets and insulin comas, even leucotomies, and in the modern day with remarkably effective phenothiazines and other anti-psychotic medications. Psychoanalysts since Sigmund Freud have tried to understand how schizophrenia affects the minds of its sufferers by communicating with what normality remains there and helping to bring self-understanding and autonomy. A combination of both approaches renders available today unprecedented potential for resolving schizophrenia in those patients who demonstrate sufficient courage and determination to adhere to a psychoanalytic psychotherapeutic treatment continuing for a number of years, and who possess sufficient patience, tolerance, forgiveness, curiosity, and generosity to be able to use their sessions fully.

In the 19th century, one view commonly held was that the concept of "unitary psychosis" included all serious mental illness. Benedict Morel in France, however, considered that mental disorders could be distinguished from each other and classified. In 1852, he observed a distinct syndrome involving withdrawal, odd mannerisms, and self-neglect which started in adolescence and led to intellectual deterioration, and he termed this "demence precoce". Further similar observations followed soon after, when Karl Kahlbaum described the condition "catatonia" in 1863 and Edwald Hecker identified a syndrome in 1871 which he termed "hebephrenia".

DOI: 10.4324/9781003433507-1

The Psychiatrist Emil Kraepelin in 1893 (Kraepelin, 1893) identified the course and symptoms of dementia praecox and distinguished it from manic-depressive psychosis, which involved primarily mood swings. Eugen Bleuler based his work (Bleuler, 1911) on Kraepelin's but was more interested in the psychological processes of dementia praecox than in the details of its symptoms; he suggested the name schizophrenia to describe what he saw as the splitting of the mind's functions. Bleuler saw "fundamental" symptoms such as disturbances of associations, changes in emotional reactions, and autism, or withdrawal from reality into an inner world of fantasy, as being distinct from "accessory" or "secondary" symptoms. These included hallucinations, delusions, catatonia or periodic states of rigidity and immobility, and other abnormal behaviours.

Contemporaneously, Sigmund Freud's view of the illness was that "the weak spot in [schizophrenic patients'] development is to be looked for somewhere between the stages of auto-erotism, narcissism and homosexuality" (Freud, 1911), indicating their sexuality's influence. He considered that in schizophrenia the patients withdraw themselves from engaging with other people (they withdraw their libido from the object) and in a narcissistic process retreat into the ego (become bound up solely in their own existence) (Freud, 1915a). Freud felt this process was so severe that in 1913 he declared that schizophrenia "is in fact incurable" (Freud, 1913). He revised this view later, in 1925 he wrote "Transference is often not so completely absent but that it can be used to a certain extent; and analysis has achieved undoubted successes with .... partial schizophrenias" (Freud, 1925). This more hopeful understanding involved the libido emerging from the ego and attaching itself in the transference (the patient's transfer of their own emotional energy onto the Psychoanalyst); the Psychoanalyst can then work directly with the patient's mind.

In the 1950s, Psychiatrist Kurt Schneider drew up a list of "first rank" symptoms of schizophrenia (Schneider, 1959), felt to be the most serious, and the clinical picture of schizophrenia was included in the International Classification of Diseases (ICD) and the Diagnostic and Statistical Manual (DSM). Several subtypes of schizophrenia were distinguished, regarding symptomatology and prognosis and therefore treatability. Historically, Karl Jaspers in 1913 contrasted "process" or endogenous schizophrenia which originates within the patient from "reactive" psychoses that develop in response to stress and have a good prognosis; that is, he made the important distinction between disease process and personality development (Jaspers, 1913). In 1933, Jacob Kasanin identified a syndrome in a group of young patients which he termed "schizoaffective disorder" that has a substantive affective component, or emotionality, a very sudden onset, and is followed by recovery (Kasanin, 1933). And subsequently, Gabriel Langfeldt distinguished schizophrenia from schizophreniform states which have a good prognosis (Langfeldt, 1939).

Thus, schizophrenia has been identified broadly as a psychotic illness, originally studied and treated by Psychiatrists but successfully addressed also, psychoanalytically, by Sigmund Freud and his followers. Melanie Klein was one of the first, followed by Freud's revised opinion in 1925, to observe both positive and negative (both warm and hostile) transference in her schizophrenic patients, with which she could therefore work in therapy with them. She indicated (Klein, 1946) the importance of paranoid and schizoid mechanisms in schizophrenic thinking, relating to suspicion and fearfulness, and schism between good and bad in the patient's relations with others. When these predominate, involving excessive projective identification (an unwanted part of the self unconsciously identifying with another person and remaining inside them) associated with persecutory anxiety and splitting, the patient's mind becomes schizoid and malfunctions. Klein also developed the concept of internal objects, where a representation of an individual's whole self may be internalised by another. Schizophrenic patients, like others, are capable of internalising their Psychoanalyst in this way.

Klein's students continued her work with schizophrenic patients. Herbert Rosenfeld described (Rosenfeld, 1947) his successful treatment of a patient, Mildred, who manifested a schizophrenic state with depersonalisation, entirely psychoanalytically when most of the analytical community of the time thought this impossible. Wilfred Bion wrote extensively about his findings while psychoanalysing schizophrenic patients. He believed that schizophrenic pathology develops as a result of poor interaction between the personality and the environment (Bion, 1967, p.37), although later he thought that physical factors might be responsible for the illness. He also concluded, confirming Melanie Klein's work, that schizophrenic patients are overly dependent on projective identification where, as described, the patient unconsciously defends their ego by sending their unpleasant and unwanted feelings into another person, perhaps from envy of them as suggested by Klein (Hinshelwood, 1989, p.179). Hanna Segal identified the phenomenon of "symbolic equation", sometimes manifest in schizophrenic patients who mistake a symbol for the real thing (Segal, 1981, p.53). Segal thinks that the symbolic equation between an original object and its symbol in the external and the internal worlds is the basis of the schizophrenic patient's concrete thinking, i.e. inability to think in abstract terms.

In North America, Heinz Hartmann (Hartmann, 1953) held that the most important defect in schizophrenia was a failure of the infant to neutralise its own aggression: though he also endorsed possible organic factors in its aetiology. Edith Jacobson, also in 1953 (Jacobson, 1953), adopted Hartmann's ego psychology approach in identifying the importance of disturbance in early ego development.

Donald Winnicott believed that schizophrenia was due to a complete absence of "good enough mothering" in early life (Winnicott, 1965b). Rosenfeld also held that schizophrenia resulted if a child experienced its mother as having a reduced tolerance of its projections towards her. Ronald Fairbairn (Fairbairn, 1954) agreed that complete maternal withdrawal leading to profound deprivation, where the infant is led to view his love as bad and destructive, could lead to schizophrenic withdrawal from emotional contact with the outside world and a highly disturbed sense of external reality. Otto Kernberg (Kernberg, 1984) theorised that psychosis was due to a blurring of boundaries between self and object representations; the child never emerges from the early symbiotic phase when his representations of himself and the object, his mother, were merged.

The interpersonal-relational approach, founded by Harry Stack Sullivan, Erich Fromm, Frieda Fromm-Reichmann, and Clara Thomson, led its contributors into active interpersonal relations with young schizophrenic people. Another interpersonalist, Harold Searles (Searles, 1963) argued that his countertransference experiences of anxiety, despair, and feeling inhuman or crazy were his schizophrenic patients' communications of childhood experiences with caregivers who had literally driven them crazy. Jay Greenberg and Stephen Mitchell's epic volume on object relations theories (Greenberg et al., 1983) usefully integrated the object relations schools with the interpersonal tradition.

Richard Lucas' book (Lucas, 2009) gives a clear account of his expertise in the management of schizophrenic patients on psychiatric wards. He, like Bion (1967, pp.43–64), Murray Jackson (2001, p.334), and Leslie Sohn (1999, p.15) understood that schizophrenic patients have both a non-psychotic and a psychotic part of their mind. When well, normal conversations are possible, but he also advocates "tuning in to the psychotic wavelength" as an additional way of engaging constructively with the patient.

Elvin Semrad, another clinician, taught Michael Robbins during the 1970s in the Massachusetts Mental Health Center, USA, to sit with schizophrenic patients during their psychoanalytic psychotherapy sessions and tolerate the burdens, conflicts, stresses and confusions, and other unimaginable states of mind besetting his patients, so that he could then, in turn, help them to bear these afflictions. Pain is subjective; but the conflictual, emotional, experiential pain of schizophrenic torment in its depth, its intensity, and its unremitting constancy during an untreated life's timeframe of years – and its effects on hope – require solid courage in both Psychoanalyst and patient in order to be tackled. Dr Michael Robbins' account of his work (Robbins, 1993) is repeatedly referred to in this volume and gives a wonderfully balanced view of the excellent psychoanalytic psychotherapy he delivered to his portfolio of 18 patients.

References

Bion, W (1967). *Second Thoughts*. pp.37, 43–64. London: Karnac.

Bleuler, E (1911). *Dementia Praecox, or the Group of Schizophrenias*. Tr. New York, 1950.

Fairbairn, R (1954). Observations on the nature of hysterical states. *British Journal of Medical Psychology*, **29**: 112–27.

Freud, S (1911). Psycho-analytic notes on an autobiographical account of a case of paranoia (Dementia Paranoides). In: *The Standard Edition of the Complete Psychological Works of Sigmund Freud*. Ed. Strachey, J. Vol. XII, p.62. London: Vintage (2001).

Freud, S (1913). The claims of psycho-analysis to scientific interest. In: *The Standard Edition of the Complete Psychological Works of Sigmund Freud*. Ed. Strachey, J. Vol. XIII, p.174. London: Vintage (2001).

Freud, S (1915a). The unconscious. In: *The Standard Edition of the Complete Psychological Works of Sigmund Freud*. Ed. Strachey, J. Vol. XIV, pp.196–7. London: Vintage (2001).

Freud, S (1925). An autobiographical study. In: *The Standard Edition of the Complete Psychological Works of Sigmund Freud*. Ed. Strachey, J. Vol. XX, p.60. London: Vintage (2001).

Greenberg, J; Mitchell, S (1983). *Object Relations in Psychoanalytic Theory*. Cambridge, MA: Harvard University Press.

Hartmann, H (1953). Contribution to the metapsychology of schizophrenia. *Psychoanalytic Study of the Child*, **8**: 177–98.

Hinshelwood, R (1989). *A Dictionary of Kleinian Thought*. p.179. London: Free Association Books.

Jackson, M (2001). *Weathering the Storms: Psychotherapy for Psychosis*. p.334. London and New York: Karnac.

Jacobson, E (1953). Contribution to the metapsychology of cyclothymic depression. In: *Affective Disorders: Psychoanalytic Contributions to Their Study*. Ed. Greenacre, P. pp.49–83. New York: International Universities Press.

Jaspers, K (1913). *Allgemeine Psychopathologie*. Springer: Berlin. *General Psychopathology*, 7th Edn. Transl. Hoenig, J; Hamilton, M. Manchester: Manchester University Press (1959).

Kasanin, J (1933). The acute schizoaffective psychoses. *American Journal of Psychiatry* (1994), **151**: 144–54.

Kernberg, O (1984). *Severe Personality Disorders: Psychotherapeutic Strategies*. New Haven, CT: Yale University Press.

Klein, M (1946). Notes on some schizoid mechanisms. In: *Envy and Gratitude and Other Works 1946–1963*. Eds. Masud, M; Khan, R. pp. 1–24. London: Hogarth Press (1984).

Kraepelin, E (1893). *Dementia Praecox and Paraphrenia*. Pub. Edinburgh: Livingstone (1919).

Langfeldt, G (1939). *The Schizophreniform States*. Copenhagen: Munksgaard.

Lucas, R (2009). *The Psychotic Wavelength*. London and New York: Routledge.

Robbins, M (1993). *Experiences of Schizophrenia: An Integration of the Personal, Scientific and Therapeutic*. New York: Guilford Press.

Rosenfeld, H (1947). Analysis of a schizophrenic state with depersonalization. *International Journal of Psychoanalysis*, **28**: 130–9.

Schneider, K (1959). *Clinical Psychopathology*. New York: Grune and Stratton.

Searles, H (1963). Transference psychosis in psychotherapy of chronic schizophrenia. In: *Collected Papers on Schizophrenia and Related Subjects (1965)*. New York: International Universities Press.

Segal, H (1981). *Delusion and Artistic Creativity & Other Psychoanalytic Essays. The Work of Hanna Segal*. p.53. London: Free Association Books.

Sohn, L (1999). Psychosis and violence. In: *Psychosis (Madness)*. Ed. Williams, P. p.15. London: Institute of Psycho-Analysis.

Winnicott, D (1965b). *The Maturational Process and the Facilitating Environment*. London: Hogarth Press.

Part I

Encountering schizophrenia

Chapter 1

Common concepts and impressions of schizophrenia

Schizophrenia is an illness that has created characteristic images in the popular mind, images that are not easy to accept. It is difficult to accept the apparent pain and disorder evident upon seeing schizophrenic individuals when we ourselves are safe and well looked after by our loved ones and friends. In the culture of today's society, schizophrenic people are outsiders, established in their lot of privation, unhappiness, often homelessness, and hopelessness. An impression of fearfulness has evolved about schizophrenia through media reports from time to time of schizophrenic patients who have attacked other people, innocent bystanders, and sometimes killed them. One of the most recent was Christopher Clunis at Finsbury Park underground station, who stabbed a man on the platform there. These reports seem to confirm in our own minds that schizophrenic patients are to be feared. In actual fact, and this is repeatedly reinforced, schizophrenic patients are usually quiet, subdued, unhappy people who would never think of attacking anybody: while the only people with whom they have a reciprocal relationship tend to be their welfare officers and clinical staff at social centres, where they receive what they need and can ask for what they see as their own solutions to their problems, sadly often only a bottle of whisky.

Distant encounters in the news

Reports in the newspapers of schizophrenic people who are paranoid create bold, frightening images of them as individuals. When a schizophrenic patient who has injured someone comes out of hospital, the headlines blazon harsh adjectives and labels referring to them which sometimes interfere with their rehabilitation in the community. And

DOI: 10.4324/9781003433507-3

when there is even a chance that we might be attacked we adhere to our own warnings on our own behalf, give schizophrenic patients a wide berth, and avoid them. They do not find it easy to approach other people calmly and according to social norms; they are clumsy, and behave inappropriately, so no one is attracted to them in order to help them, and they remain isolated from the public. But assessments in hospital ensure that their illness is under control, so that upon release they are managed through appointments with staff at regular intervals. Personal reactions to them among the public, however, are commonly to shun them and jeer and persecute them rather than to see that they are ill and doing their best to conform to the arrangements made for them.

Paranoid schizophrenia is a potentially dangerous condition, but the danger is rare since patients who suffer from it tend to be picked up within the mental health system with psychological symptoms long before they physically harm anyone. Mental health staff are skilled at treating them and are capable of spotting signs that indicate they still require treatment and careful management. If they are a danger to others, they are removed to a special hospital and looked after by specialist staff. Paranoid schizophrenia usually affects the patient by making them wary of other people and causing them to keep themselves to themselves, away from others. But newspaper headlines reinforce the idea that they are a danger to the public, and the prejudice continues to be believed and adhered to.

Many of the destitute in the streets are schizophrenic patients. They tend to be dishevelled and disorganised individuals familiar to most of us as we live our daily lives. The common conception we hold of them is generally accurate regarding the truth of how they live. We tend to give them a wide berth and be wary of them, when the truth that we all really do know about them is that they are suffering, probably all too aware in many ways of their predicament, and struggling to survive within the means they have to help themselves. The health service ensures that each such patient who comes to their attention knows where they should go to find help when they think they need it. The patients wander about on the streets rather than staying in sheltered accommodation where they could keep clean and care for themselves properly; it is commonly their decision to leave the security of these centres and expose themselves to the consequent dangers. The public is faced with their seemingly hopeless plight without being able to help them. This in itself is painful, and therefore the public can unconsciously feel resentful that these destitute people do not respond more fully to the help they are supplied with. The public, in fact, sometimes needs reassurance, for example, at Christmas time, that the destitute wandering the streets are being helped; we find it hard to believe that anyone could choose to live like this rather than in clean, secure accommodation. The public can even feel a level of resentment towards them for upsetting their peace and happiness at Christmas time. Schizophrenia prevents the thinking that might allow them to conform, and this adds through their consequent behaviour to the public's image of unkempt, unreachable strangers whom they do not want to meet.

These behaviours of schizophrenic patients are due to their illness' effect on their minds. The prevailing experience a schizophrenic patient lives through seems to be one of total meaninglessness, created in their minds by the overwhelming factors underlying schizophrenia: not enough warmth, no evident meaning to be found anywhere, and total lack of hope. Their mental outlook is bleak. They are unable to arrange better circumstances for themselves because they choose a peripatetic existence, wandering around, rather than settling down and trying to live an ordered life. They rarely have reliable contacts with whom they could share a friendly conversation, a cup of coffee, or accommodation. Their attention span is short; their minds flit and do not settle so as to develop any kind of plan or structured existence. They may appear interested in the people around them, but this is usually only to enquire about the accessibility of alcohol, drugs, or money for their perceived future of the next hour or two. Beyond that, their view appears to be entirely vacuous. Their illness is entirely entrenched within their mind; the window within which beneficial treatment could have been started has long since passed. Commonly starting in early adult life, this is the age at which psychoanalytic psychotherapy is most effective; but by the time the patient has become a vagrant, very little intervention into their mind is possible. They remain dissolute, disordered, and beyond the possibility of psychotherapy and certainly any psychoanalytic interventions of any kind.

Close encounters with schizophrenic strangers

Schizophrenic patients often look rather different from normal. They may be untidy or dishevelled, and they may move about as if in their own world, entirely detached from other people around them. Their different appearance makes us feel uneasy, and commonly concerned about them, and about ourselves in relation to them.

It is a tendency of human nature to think that what is different from ourselves is dangerous. We fear people who look out of place in the environment where we ourselves are wondering why they are there, and what it is about them that makes them behave so differently from ourselves.

But schizophrenic patients are rarely dangerous. It is only if the patient feels so badly treated themselves, and consequently vulnerable, that they believe they must defend themselves. This experience of fear that they carry is what lies behind an attack that, rarely, they might make on another person. It is very rarely that this happens; mostly the patient is sad and lonely and simply trying to survive as best they can, though in their primitive and very inept way.

A lack of identity leads to the patient wandering about aimlessly, as we often see them in the street. Lack of an identity based on reality or, indeed, a misguided sense of identity, is also found in schizophrenic patients who are confident but entirely unrealistic and mistaken in what they think. These patients can sometimes be difficult to identify as schizophrenic, as they may keep their mistaken ideas well hidden in their psyche and only rarely act on them. Fortunately, however, they are rarely actually dangerous.

Schizophrenic patients have developed a system of thinking that is not in accordance with the real world, i.e. they relate through their own system to the real world. The patient particularly manifests overt illness and experiences pain at the boundaries between these two worlds. Sometimes there is more than one "world" in addition to reality. Therapy tries to make inroads into their unreal worlds and show the patient where they are mistaken.

It is the usual finding that once youth has passed, these patients are very hard for therapists and clinicians to treat. Their minds have become largely stabilised, or indeed entrenched, into questionable habitual attitudes and incorrect assumptions that no one can disabuse them of. They live according to these mistaken ideas and find learning anything else extremely difficult. The schizophrenic process by middle age has done its worst, and the patients generally do not live much beyond this due to difficulty in monitoring their physical health. Social centres aim to check regularly their physical parameters, but the patients tend towards vagrancy, and attending recalls for health checks is not high on their list of priorities.

The different parts of a schizophrenic patient's mind do not connect together with each other, as would be required for mental health.

Parts of their mind are linked with experiences they have had in different parts of their known environments. These islands of awareness become largely lost to them because their essential self is not fully established. They are not able to locate these experiences in their mind when something stimulates memorable aspects of them, a fleeting memory which they cannot place in context. This detached nature of accumulated experiences gained throughout their life lies behind their confusion. They become more and more confused and unable to help themselves. They hanker more and more for an experience of life once known to them, living in the past, but are less and less able to live in the present. They cannot draw on stable relations with their environment because of their lack of representation of helpful sources of sustenance in their mind; they commonly cannot take full advantage of the resources provided for them in their social centre. Dementia as well as schizophrenia takes its toll on the lives of these unfortunate individuals. Their healthcare is striven for, but their life expectancy is around 20 years shorter than for the mentally healthier majority of the population.

Schizophrenic patients sometimes have a very human aspect that part of them which has taken in the normal, real world and has responded to it. This part of them can engage with other people while they ignore as well as they can the part of themselves that has been damaged by pain and that they themselves have to tolerate. It is this dichotomy that causes them to have a "split mind", and be "schizophrenic"; but while they are able and can be encouraged to live in the well, happy part of their mind, these patients can be lively, engaging and friendly, often gentle souls, with feelings like non-schizophrenic people. Approaching them with kindness brings out the best in them, as in us all.

"It's schizophrenic" is not a respectful and therefore not an acceptable way to use the word "schizophrenic". "Schizophrenic" means "split mind", and only people have minds. People are schizophrenic if they are unfortunate enough to have found themselves thinking the unthinkable over periods of time in their young lives when they did not have access to psychological comfort. These experiences were, for them, extraordinarily painful. The patients who are schizophrenic therefore deserve respect and compassion for their distress, and plays and situations preferably discussed as conflicted, with divided opinions and contradictory feelings and issues, rather than "schizophrenic".

Relating to schizophrenic friends and family members

Schizophrenic members of the family are usually singled out as being "different" from the other family members. It may be difficult to understand them, while they may not understand the other family members. They may be poorly functioning individuals, socially, at work, and regarding their own personal hygiene. Occasionally hostility is expressed, although more commonly the situation is that ill-feeling is surfacing due to the family's predicament. A parent with schizophrenia may present very real difficulties for their spouse and especially for any children they may have. Almost certainly, the social services will be involved with the family, to safeguard its cohesion despite the influence of the ill member, to restore harmony and wellbeing as far as possible, and to oversee the progress of the children as they try to grow up with the least adverse effects from the illness in the family as possible.

Schizophrenic individuals may have been friends with others before their schizophrenia became apparent. Nearly always they will have been quiet, friendly, gentle people, for whom all their friends will have been very saddened indeed at their demise. Perhaps they will have been childhood friends, whose sad lapse into illness has been accompanied by growth and development into health of their neighbours and siblings. Friendship is highly valued by schizophrenic people who once were highly functioning, intelligent individuals who appreciated life, as did Sir Aubrey Lewis' suffering young man with negative symptoms (see Chapter 3). Genuine, concerned friends who shared experiences such as university life may visit a sick friend in hospital, which the schizophrenic patient will greatly value and is certainly preventive regarding suicide.

The Psychoanalyst's regard for his patient

It was finally agreed by Freud, especially when Melanie Klein had made her findings clear, that schizophrenic patients may indeed be psychoanalysed. Klein had some success, especially with children in her care, and Herbert Rosenfeld demonstrated that a patient may be psychoanalysed by psychoanalytic technique only, when this was considered impossible.

As Dr Michael Robbins found and wrote about in his clinical reports (Robbins, 1993), transference is necessary by the schizophrenic patient onto the Psychoanalyst no less than for any other psychoanalytic treatment. His patient Sara (Robbins, 2012) was slightly unkempt and "of odd appearance", but he detected transference from her, and so was able to deliver her treatment of psychoanalytic psychotherapy.

Psychoanalytically, encounters with schizophrenic patients concern the calm, reflective psychoanalytic mind as much as they bewilder the normal mind. But a medically qualified, Psychiatry-trained Psychoanalyst is trained to make sense of the patient's schizophrenia; he recognises much of what she manifests in terms of her appearance; the tone of her communications; sometimes – from what has gone before – what she invisibly, unconsciously relates to in her mind and is fearful of; and what she is mistakenly thinking, perhaps expressed as delusions or thought disorder (see Chapters 3 and 6). The Psychiatry-trained Psychoanalyst is able to recognise frank psychosis in her, but also to detect elements of her personality, feelings, and characteristics, especially as time proceeds and he becomes more familiar with her tendencies. He is able to help her to communicate with him what she is thinking, and especially what she would say if she were not prevented from doing so by psychological factors which the Psychoanalyst is trained to detect. He helps her externalise her thoughts and feelings and brings her into experiencing herself and the world around her in good relation to reality, whereas previously she was bound up in her own, usually very unpleasant, experience which did not reflect reality except the unpleasant reality which was originally familiar to her; in doing so, he helps her resolve her schizophrenia.

References

Robbins, M (1993). *Experiences of Schizophrenia: An Integration of the Personal, Scientific and Therapeutic*. New York: Guilford Press.

Robbins, M (2012). The successful psychoanalytic therapy of a schizophrenic woman. *Psychodynamic Psychiatry*, **40**(4): 575–608.

Daily newspapers.

Television news and documentary reporting.

Chapter 2

Schizophrenia in families

Schizophrenia tends to run in families. But there is no single gene which is responsible for schizophrenia in an individual, and the genetic causes remain unclear. Having a parent or a brother or sister with schizophrenia increases the risk, as does brain injury around the time of birth and the increasing age of the father. An identical twin of a schizophrenic patient will have a genetic predisposition towards a 1 in 2 chance of developing the illness. Genes and the family environment both play a part in an individual's likelihood of becoming schizophrenic. The two factors combine to increase the risk, and genes can affect the brain or behaviour in families to increase the risk for a person becoming schizophrenic. It is sometimes quite painful to relate to a family member who is afflicted with schizophrenia. In some families they are much loved and can be a focus of family affection; whereas if they are a parent, family arrangements can become quite difficult for other members of the family. The spouse of a schizophrenic member may have a challenging role in managing their husband's or wife's vulnerability as well as looking after any children of the family. Schizophrenic children usually require special schooling.

Parents as schizophrenic patients

If a patient is well managed by healthcare or social workers then their family's life may continue relatively smoothly. Enabling a parent to enjoy free expression and a comfortable latitude to their behaviour must be counterbalanced by their effects on the people around them. They may be able to undertake minor responsibilities, including in relation to their children, but overall are dependent on their spouse to make arrangements that affect the family as a whole. The family's

DOI: 10.4324/9781003433507-4

attitudes to them are likely to fluctuate depending on how much disruption is associated with their illness; children may learn to accept that this parent is 'different' from other people. If there is more than one adult with schizophrenia in the extended family, the family members may be familiar with this situation and adjust accordingly. Parents with established schizophrenia are not suitable for psychoanalytic psychotherapy because of its stresses, but rather for supportive psychotherapy if this is found to help them, and social supervision.

Schizophrenic patients can internalise loved people as good internal objects, like healthy people, once their ego has been strengthened and its boundaries established. When a patient has adjusted to the realities of herself and the world around her, the environments she moves in and the people she meets, she may prove sociable and make close friends. Reaching this state from her earlier condition of schizophrenic illness, through psychoanalytic psychotherapy, may only gradually develop, however, and not all patients are able to withstand the demands and rigours of a psychoanalytic psychotherapeutic treatment in order fully to achieve it. For those who can reach this experience, however, their rewards and benefits may be valued for the rest of their lives.

Schizophrenic children

Childhood schizophrenia is not common, but children of a schizophrenic parent and children who go on to develop schizophrenia tend to show slow development in motor skills, lack of engagement with other people, and withdrawal rather than an outgoing nature. Their cognitive development is often restricted and their educational attainment is less than average. In the family, they may be overlooked or ignored due to their lack of engagement. The early stages of "negative" schizophrenia are characterised by increasing lethargy, inertia, and disinterest as the child grows older. Psychiatric intervention may result in medication administration, but possibilities for restoring the child to normal liveliness are limited.

If a young person shows signs of serious distress or developing symptoms of isolating and concerning behaviour, an assessment consultation may be needed with an early intervention Psychiatry team from the local hospital. In very mild cases, this may be all that is required to calm or settle the young person regarding his or her concerns. Medication may be provided, to be taken for several months at least, and a follow-up appointment to establish how well the patient has become able to manage themselves. Accommodation in a hospital ward is becoming increasingly scarce, even for patients who might feel safer there, and sometimes to the concern of their parents who may feel very anxious about continuing to supervise their offspring at home. If the patient is seriously ill, a bed may be found at a distance from their home, which, again, is not ideal. But medications can help a patient to feel calmer, and if the intervention interview has gone well and explanations are offered, with reassurance and follow-up by the same doctor, the young person may feel cared for sufficiently to carry on at home as before. In cases of serious, psychotic illness, if a thera-pist is available the young person may be accepted for treatment when they have stabilised and begin a long course of therapy, with carefully prescribed medication. This can be expensive, so not all of those who could benefit from it will be able to do so. A shorter form of supportive psychotherapy is likely to help those with less serious illness, often in combination with medication. Parents like to know their offspring will recover, and the patient may be under a lot of pressure to "get well". The parents will almost certainly be very concerned if a diagnosis of schizophrenia is eventually made. They need to be informed about what this will entail and supported until they become able to care for the young person within the family.

For a schizophrenic patient within their family, their sadness and deeply unpleasant experience can be very hard to tolerate. If diag-nosed, they will be on medication which, it is hoped, will take away the "edge" of their symptoms though they may not themselves be aware of this. Siblings, any brothers or sisters, may not be patient with them and may be quite unkind. Alternatively, in a loving fam-ily, they may settle into their "niche" but still have to cope with their unpleasant experiences. As they grow older, employment may offer opportunities to meet other people and mix, especially in sheltered employment, so that any skills they may have could come to the fore. A loving family makes a big difference to them, though they may not know anything different; but a patient in an uncaring family lives a much harsher life.

Financial effects

A schizophrenic member brings financial realities to their family that must be addressed. A mean of 5.6 hours of support per day is given to schizophrenic patients, which is equivalent to £34,000 per person with schizophrenia being cared for by a family member per year (Manga-lore et al., 2007). As mentioned, schizophrenic patients who wish to and are able to work can be found sheltered employment; this contrib-utes to the family income and is good for the patient who may enjoy a consequent degree of independence and validated autonomy through doing this. Work colleagues, aware of this arrangement, usually ac-commodate the schizophrenic partner with good spirit and work along-side him or her without any problems.

Practical aspects of understanding psychosis

Current psychological understanding holds that psychosis is the re-sult of the unconscious mind defending itself through entirely un-realistic means from unpleasant, undesirable, or harmful ideas that it has been presented with and has tried to internalise. It may also be viewed as the output of a brain compromised by physiological disturbance.

Entirely unrealistic or inappropriate aspects of appearance, thought, or behaviour become manifest in a patient who is psychotic. The unconscious defence mechanisms of psychosis lead to unrealis-tic language and behaviour, and so do not conform to the reality of the real world around the patient; she appears "out of kilter", "out of sync", "odd", and evidently not mentally well even to the untrained observer.

The patient, or her relatives, will be keen to find a therapist who can "make her well again". A psychotic patient must be treated by a doctor who is trained in the understanding and management of psycho-sis: a Psychiatrist. Psychiatrists almost always prescribe anti-psychotic medication to a psychotic patient because it is kind to relieve her of her mistaken thinking, to encourage her thoughts to return to the real world. It would be best for the Psychiatrist also, first, to note and to try to listen and make psychodynamic sense of what the patient says while she is psychotic, so that the truths of the ideas behind these psychotic defence mechanism-based words may later be addressed (see Chapter 6). The ideas that have actually and basically disturbed her will under-lie her evident, mad, psychotic presentation. If the Psychiatrist could do this, the patient's progress in hospital would actually bring about some healing for the patient through correcting something in her life that her mind has found too difficult to internalise. These days psy-chotic defence mechanisms, studied as psychodynamics, are quite well understood and so could be utilised to understand each newly admitted psychotic patient.

Schizophrenia is one form of psychosis. Psychosis, being the result of unrealistic defence mechanisms protecting the mind from unwanted or painful ideas, can be a part of a number of separate illnesses. It may be an emotionally based disorder accompanied by disturbed cognition, in schizoaffective disorder. It may be a direct consequence of very disturbed emotion, as in psychotic depression or in mania. It may occur during fluctuating emotion so severe as to disturb the perception of reality, as in bipolar disorder. Sometimes the term "psychotic" is used simply to refer to the condition of patients who are out of touch with reality. It can be used to represent schizophrenia, with all the concomitants of this diagnosis (see Chapter 3) but really should not, academically, because as seen above the term can apply to other psychotic illnesses.

The features of psychosis differ from patient to patient and depend on the nature and diagnosis of the underlying illness. Schizophrenic psychosis is believed to be caused by an excess of the neurotransmitter dopamine in the brain, since drugs that stabilise psychotic schizophrenic patients such as phenothiazines or newer antipsychotic medications all oppose dopamine production. The psychotic symptoms of schizophrenia and the experiences of living with it are described in Chapter 3. Manic psychosis is characterised by flights of often-grandiose ideas, and depressive psychosis by intense rumination, with the patient turning over the same sad, doleful thoughts again and again in their mind, often accompanied by anxiety. Bipolar psychosis involves sudden mood swings from being highly elated with expansive statements and overactivity, as in mania, to deep depression that can be stultifying. Psychosis implies that the patient is out of touch with reality, and all these symptoms indicate the wide range of ways that psychosis can affect patients.

Psychosis is a severe affliction which should be treated as soon as it is recognised in a patient and the nature of the patient's predicament has been established as far as possible. Early intervention services aim to establish as clearly as possible the nature of a young person's difficulties surrounding their demise by talking with them and encouraging them to outline their needs. Details of what they say are recorded so that at a later date their issues may be examined more closely and rectified if this can be arranged; psychodynamic scrutiny can reveal helpful aspects to the intervention service's clinicians. Psychotic individuals are very vulnerable since they are not in touch with the reality around them. They require to be cared for by relatives or, if this cannot be done, then to be taken to a place of safety until they recover or to a hospital if a place can be found for them to be treated. There is currently a great shortage of hospital beds for such patients, who sometimes are provided for only at a considerable distance from their homes. Psychiatrists, like all health service staff, work extremely hard to provide a good service for all who need it and recognise that psychotic patients are among the most needful of all their mentally ill patients. The cognitive confusion of schizophrenia may be the most debilitating of symptoms, but mood disorders such as mania and deep depression also require very careful management.

As has been discussed for schizophrenia, psychosis is a state of mind which is only very rarely dangerous towards other people. The sufferer is out of touch with reality, and so their mind moves among ideas which are unrealistic but not necessarily harmful at all to others. The clinical staff treating and managing them will know their precise diagnosis and will treat their psychosis accordingly. While the patient is clinically psychotic, he or she may not be in a state to communicate in any readily understandable way with other people; but once in a more stable state, they may be grateful for company. It is difficult to work out what a psychotic patient is thinking while the psychosis lasts; clinicians skilled in psychodynamic therapy may make sense of some aspects of the patient's words, but they, too, have to wait until the patient is speaking rationally to understand how they can help them best. If there is any sign of violence the patient's management changes accordingly, so that the staff and anyone else in contact with the patient are afforded protection. Proportionately few patients demonstrate violence, however; when newly taken ill, the majority are predominantly distressed by their own psychosis. This may, however, lead to physical disturbance later on. It is very rare for a member of the public to experience violence from a hospital patient; hospital management is generally very effective in Britain. Supportive psychotherapy is found to be helpful for even psychotic patients when they have returned to non-psychotic thinking; this helps them to adjust towards normality rather than suffering in their psychotic world. Psychoanalytic psychotherapy is a major undertaking which only a few suitable patients are usually assessed for, and this tends to be started following an interval after their hospitalisation when they have stabilised from their illness. All too many patients find managing their schizophrenia too great an ordeal, resulting in their consequent suicide.

Reference

Mangalore, R; Knapp, M (2007). Cost of schizophrenia in England. *Journal of Mental Health Policy and Economics*, **10**(1): 23–41.

Chapter 3

The observed and the experiential faces of schizophrenia

The appearance of schizophrenia in a person takes a different form for each patient, creates deep uncertainty for their friends and relatives, and is profoundly worrying and upsetting for everyone. The medical doctors who treat patients with it, Psychiatrists, need to be clear whether their patient has it or not so they know what treatment to provide for them. They regard their patient as an individual, but also observe them carefully to see whether they manifest or not the exact symptom details included in a list which defines the illness "schizophrenia". Specific, experienced symptoms of schizophrenia may be considered as subsumed into the general experience of the illness. By all accounts, this is extremely unpleasant. The numbness of endogenous and negative schizophrenia, which may be experienced at times also in reactive schizophrenia, prevents enactment of thoughts and ideas the patient may have. The environmentally reactive patient, by contrast, is likely to enact very actively what occurs to them as they experience their increasing and most unwelcome symptoms, of which they will be acutely aware.

Schizophrenia observed

The observed signs of schizophrenia provide Psychiatrists with the criteria necessary to determine the diagnosis of schizophrenia and its treatment. Kurt Schneider identified eight "first rank" symptoms, which are rarely found in other disorders and therefore have a major role in the contemporary diagnosis of schizophrenia, although Schneider's view in 1959 was that they are neither necessary nor sufficient for the diagnosis (Gelder, Harrison and Cowen, 2006, p.275). Hearing thoughts spoken aloud and descriptive auditory hallucinations about

DOI: 10.4324/9781003433507-5

the patient are two first-rank symptoms. Hallucinations in the form of an audible commentary on the patient's activities, or relating to the body, are also included in this group. Thought withdrawal from or insertion into the patient's mind, or being broadcast, i.e. being spoken aloud are further forms of thought disorder almost exclusively found in schizophrenia. Delusional perceptions, i.e. reaching a false conclusion as a result of a perception, or feelings or actions experienced as made or influenced by external agents are additional unusual symptoms which are rarely found in any but schizophrenic patients.

It is combinations of criteria provided in the Diagnostic Criteria from DSM-5-TR ™ (DSM-5-TR™, 2022) which is used in the USA, and in the ICD-10 Classification of Mental and Behavioural Disorders (ICD-10, 1994), used in Europe and elsewhere, which define schizophrenia for diagnostic purposes. The two systems have much in common regarding their main features, but differ in some of the detail, having been developed on different continents.

The ICD-10 holds, in summary, that the normal requirement for a diagnosis of schizophrenia is that:

a minimum of one very clear symptom (and usually two or more if less clear-cut) belonging to any one of the following groups must be apparent for at least one month:

- Thoughts echoing in the patient's mind, thought insertion or withdrawal; thought broadcasting
- Delusions of control, influence, or being acted upon clearly referred to the body or limb movements, or to specific thoughts, actions, or sensations; or delusional perceptions
- Hallucinatory voices giving a running commentary on the patient's behaviour, or discussing the patient among themselves, or other types of hallucinatory voices
- Persistent delusions that are culturally inappropriate and completely impossible

or:

symptoms from at least two of the following groups must be apparent for at least one month:

- Persistent audible, visible, or physically felt hallucinations
- Breaks or interjections in the train of thought, resulting in incoherent or irrelevant speech, or made-up words

- Bizarre behaviour such as physical excitement, posturing, having malleable limbs which retain their manipulated position, or resisting suggestions and doing the opposite; inability to speak; lethargy
- Negative" symptoms such as marked apathy; poverty of speech; blunt or incongruous emotional responses
- A significant and consistent change in the overall quality of some aspects of personal behaviour, manifest as loss of interest, aimlessness, idleness, a self-absorbed attitude, and social withdrawal

(ICD-10)

(Copyright Elsevier)

The DSM-5-TR™ indicates similar priorities for the diagnostic symptoms of schizophrenia, as a separate authority used in the USA.

Hallucinations, delusions, and disorders of active thought, speech, and movement have been described as "positive" symptoms of schizophrenia which are abnormal when present. The "negative" features referred to, including stultification, a stolid appearance, and apparent lack of thought, emotion, or activity are abnormal by their absence and were distinguished from the "positive" features by Tim Crow (Crow, 1980). From this, he proposed two syndromes of schizophrenia: Type I, characterised by the predominance of positive symptoms and due to an overactivity of the brain's dopaminergic system; the other, Type II, showing predominantly negative symptoms, and due to cellular loss in the brain structures, as being part of the same disease. The relative prevalence of positive and negative aspects of a patient's presentation has a bearing on their prognosis and treatability: negative features augur less well for the patient.

Peter Liddle in 1987 (Liddle, 1987), using cluster analysis, identified in place of Crow's two categories, three clusters of signs and symptoms: two clusters of positive symptoms, the "reality distortion" syndrome, comprising hallucinations and delusions and sometimes paranoia, typical of psychosis, indicating the patient is out of touch with reality, and the "disorganization" syndrome, including incoherent speech and inappropriate emotional responses; and a third "psychomotor poverty" syndrome involving poverty of speech, poverty of action, and blunted emotions, all negative features. These three clusters have been replicated in several further studies, indicating coherence in some way as yet unknown of how schizophrenic patients' minds are impaired by their illness.

The previously widely adopted distinction between "acute" and "chronic" regarding the different patterns of relapse and remission seen in schizophrenia, and from this the nature of illness experienced, has now been superseded in its usefulness by consideration of a patient's risk factors; the more severe and the greater the number of these, the more entirely will the patient's life be affected by the illness, in time and in extent and in nature.

Genetic inheritance, as indicated likely by a clear family history of the illness, suggests a "process" kind of illness which develops insidiously through life, endogenously based within the patient. An absence of family history and the presence of trauma or adverse circumstances make an illness more likely to be a more treatable "reactive" one, with consequently a much better prognosis. Positive rather than negative symptoms, female gender, adult onset rather than in childhood, a definite affective component, and a short duration of untreated psychosis between onset and commencement of treatment all improve the possibility of a good outcome.

The disease process of schizophrenia is not well understood except for evidence of abnormally active dopamine pathways, including especially the mesolimbic pathway, together with abnormal dopamine receptors in the nucleus accumbens and compromised prefrontal lobe function, and widespread degeneration of brain tissue. "Schizophrenia" may be a continuum between an insidiously pathological brain syndrome and, as Elvin Semrad put it, an individual's "sacrifice of reality to preserve life" when his or her environment is intolerable to themselves (Robbins, 1993, p.172). As mentioned in the Historical Review herein, and again above, Karl Jaspers distinguished between endogenous schizophrenia and reactive psychoses, thus indicating the important difference between disease process and personality development. If this difference could be ascertained clinically during selection of patients for psychoanalytic psychotherapy, from levels of alertness and other signs in the patient, then those patients deemed suitable could be chosen with a greater degree of confidence.

Schizophrenia may affect people of any age, with the age of onset varying from childhood to past middle age, although ages 15–54 are the ages of incidence most commonly seen. Between the ages of 20–24 both men's and women's incidence peaks markedly, men more so than women, though after the age of 35 women outnumber men.

The role of affect in the symptomatology of a schizophrenic patient is important as a guide to their prognosis. A significant affective component, where definite emotional elements are seen, suggests much better progress might be possible than if little affective change is observed. As with positive symptoms contrasted with negative symptoms, and an evident reactive component in an illness contrasted with its insidious progress from infancy onwards, manifest emotion is to be welcomed as a sign of hope for the patient. And the best time to start treating a patient, even if only with a consultation and medication, is before the duration of untreated psychosis has extended for too long, i.e. while the personality is still largely intact. An acute illness, presenting with a sudden onset in a bright, lively, intelligent patient, has a much better prognosis than is indicated by an insidiously developing illness; and unlike those with an illness of gradual onset, such a patient may respond well to psychotherapy.

While the illness "schizophrenia" may thus be considered internally somewhat heterogeneous, there are also several related illnesses which must be separated from it diagnostically for purposes of prognostic assessment and effective treatment.

Paranoid schizophrenia, specified as an individual illness in the ICD-10, remains the most treatable form of schizophrenia. Schizoaffective disorder, identified in both DSM-5-TR™ and ICD-10 as a diagnosis which includes schizophrenic, depressive, and sometimes also manic symptoms in its presentation, has a good prognosis when treated. Schizophreniform disorder, which is also specified as a discrete diagnosis in DSM-5-TR™, is a transient psychosis which may go on to develop into full-blown schizophrenia, affective disorder, or schizoaffective disorder. There is evidence for some genetic overlap between all these diagnoses, and also with schizotypal personality disorder which, however, is not treatable with psychoanalytic psychotherapy; some genes are even shared with bipolar disorder. Several shared genes have been implicated in their common genetic inheritance, but the importance of this is that some patients with schizoid illness are genetically afflicted with an inherited, developmental illness which is not treatable by psychoanalytic psychotherapy, while others also have the genetic complement but have spontaneously reacted to adverse circumstances, and may be helped to resolve their illness through treatment. Accurate diagnosis therefore indicates among which forms of psychotic illness likely patients suitable for psychoanalytic psychotherapy are to be found. The individual patient's accessibility during interview, her aptitude for transference, and any clear history of earlier personal application and good character can indicate when there is a real opportunity for a successful psychoanalytic psychotherapeutic treatment outcome.

The patient's experience of schizophrenia

Before the advent of effective medications, the physicians Philippe Pinel and John Haslam, both writing independently, in 1809, wrote the first authentic accounts of schizophrenia. Observing his patients experiencing its effects, Haslam noted its negative aspects and cases occurring in young people, two areas of particular concern today.

Sir Aubrey Lewis in 1967 quoted a particularly memorable account by a boy of 18 years who had been ill for at least a year:

> I am more and more losing contact with my environment and with myself. Instead of taking an interest in what goes on and caring about what happens with my illness, I am all the time losing my emotional contact with everything including myself. What remains is only an abstract knowledge of what goes on around me and of the internal happenings in myself.... Even this illness which pierces to the centre of my whole life I can regard only objectively. But, on rare occasions, I am overwhelmed with the sudden realisation of the ghastly destruction that is caused by this creeping uncanny disease that I have fallen a victim to.... My despair sometimes floods over me. But after each such outburst I become more indifferent, I lose myself more in the disease, I sink into an almost oblivious existence. My fate when I reflect upon it is the most horrible one can conceive of. I cannot picture anything more frightful than for a well-endowed cultivated human being to live through his own gradual deterioration fully aware of it all the time. But that is what is happening to me.
>
> (Lewis, 1967, pp. 16–29)
> (Reproduced by permission of Taylor and Francis Group)

This terrible account is notable because it outlines the negative aspects of schizophrenia, which are much less well recorded in the literature from the patient's perspective than the positive syndrome involving hallucinations and delusions and positive thought disorder. It also seems to be endogenous, since he does not complain of any aspect of the reality around himself.

Dr Michael Robbins' description of a patient, Sara, conveys much of what her unhappy experience apparently consisted of, in terms of positive symptoms of schizophrenia:

> She was drab, overweight, dressed in baggy clothing and the general impression she conveyed was one of indeterminate gender.

Her gaze was vacant .... and her discourse was vague. Although she claimed to be nervous she gave little outward evidence. I learned from the hospital psychiatrist that she spent long periods of time huddled in corners, mute and rigid except for bizarre facial expressions, but all Sara told me was that her problem was inability to concentrate and lack of a sense of personal identity...

During our appointments Sara would sit near the door with her head averted, often with her coat on and purse clutched to her lap; and she often bolted out the door a few minutes early. Her posture was rigid and her gestures and facial expressions were contorted and contextually inappropriate. She was detached, her voice was flat, whispery, and without affect and she did not make eye contact. There were long silences sometimes punctuated with sotto voce mocking laughter or muttered curses or gibberish about shapes and patterns. She had auditory and visual hallucinations. She believed bombs were planted in the walls and planes and missiles were about to attack and kill her.

(Robbins, 2012, pp.578–9)
(Reprinted with permission of Dr Michael
Robbins and Guilford Press)

Dr Robbins had recognised Sara's intelligence and wide vocabulary, and in view of this sat with her, responding to her utterances, until her ability to think despite her symptoms enabled her to communicate meaningfully with him, and Dr Robbins to help her to clarify her utter confusion. Sitting patiently with patients while they learned to do this was a skill that Elvin Semrad showed him and his colleagues while in training.

Elvin Semrad, Michael Robbins' mentor from the Massachusetts Mental Health Center, USA, maintained that schizophrenia is "the sacrifice of reality to preserve life, or for purposes of survival", implying a reality not worth preserving by the patient. It would seem apparent that this situation for a patient, a need to sacrifice reality, is slightly different from that of the very unfortunate young man's case quoted above, suffering from negative symptoms, who had no complaints about external reality or other people but only about the slow, insidious degeneration of his life. The young man in this account is, however, an example in its early stages of the dreadful definition of a patient who suffers the insidious and negative aspects of endogenous schizophrenia as being "barely conscious when perfectly wakeful". This poor young man would seem to be moving in this dire direction.

Severely ill patients with advanced endogenous or process schizophrenia, and especially those with the negative syndrome, appear to be "ground down" and subdued by their suffering, while reactive patients who have been subject in the past to trauma or other unpleasant experiences may be quite aware that "something is wrong" and painfully alert in response to this, possibly due to the stimulation of what is being reacted to.

Endogenous schizophrenia in its early stages begins so insidiously that the patient may not be specifically aware of their illness. Awareness of all forms of the illness is probably greatest when its early stages have an impact on a generally healthy mind. If a patient presents with a reactive illness, aware of their unpleasant experience of a world intolerable to them, they might have a chance of stabilising in the reality of the real world. This would be the reactive patient's opportunity for psychoanalytic psychotherapy, if only it could be offered to them. The poor young man's endogenously collapsing inner world would today be best helped by the most effective contemporary medications and all support and care.

In younger patients with reactive or milder forms of illness such as paranoid schizophrenia or schizoaffective disorder, around the time of onset, they may be vociferous and excitable and express an intense desire to find help. They may be very keen to talk to their early intervention service clinician; their families may be equally needing support and reassurance on their behalf. The duration of untreated psychosis, the interval between onset of symptoms and receiving treatment, should be kept to an absolute minimum, to preserve the personality as far as possible; it is extremely important to try to preserve their premorbid personality despite the symptoms during the ensuing weeks and months, albeit while taking necessary antipsychotic medication; some preparations are not markedly sedative and can be very helpful in allowing the patient to continue functioning normally. Through consultation and administering some medication, the young patient may be stabilised; although alleviating their experience of the environment where the psychosis developed is unfortunately not always possible. Subsequent follow-up observation is indicated, however, to establish accurate diagnosis and scope for psychological treatment.

Some aspects of the experience of schizophrenia may be common to both positive and negative illness syndromes. Bewilderment and perplexity at the circumstance that has befallen the patient are very common. They cannot understand themselves. They are dependent on others for simple decisions and sometimes basic help when they cannot fend for themselves. Their autonomy has vanished. Their studies or work is a terrible effort and they cannot fathom why this should be so. At the onset of symptoms that cannot be overlooked, a young person is commonly determined to get themselves out of this situation; this healthy streak in their personality should be carefully protected until their time of psychological therapy, when it will be essential for pulling them through their difficulties and out into better life.

Anxiety, wariness of others, and frank fear at times about their present situation or the future may grip the patient. In cases where abuse has occurred much effort may be made by the offender to disguise or deny this, but strong negative affect towards a member of the family should always be noted and discussed with the patient. Fearful hallucinations or delusions experienced by the patient should be treated with medication after any available sense concerning them has been elicited from the patient. Kindly conversation can reassure them, but the fearful experiences will become memories which will have to be discussed in therapy when the patient is ready. Human contact can be comforting on a psychiatric ward, and advice given to supportive family members to remind them to be gentle in exchanges with their ill relatives.

Spontaneous affect breakdown can disturb family members, who cannot understand it. Even if the patient's illness does not have a large affective component, "irrational" anger, actually precipitated by a sense of injustice in the unavoidable presence of an abuser when everyone else is unaware of the truth, should alert the clinician. All care needs to be taken to ensure the patient understands that physical aggression or violence is completely unacceptable, but talking through the patient's feelings with them may defuse some of the force they are trying to vent.

Misery, and secondary or "post-schizophrenic" depression, are very common, and if marked may be treated with antidepressants. Keeping the patient in touch with others nearby, with occupational therapy if they are in hospital, or other distracting activities, may lighten their experience for some of the time. Persuading them to verbalise their feelings can help to put these in perspective, but the seriousness of their condition is not easy to ameliorate. Suicidal thoughts must always be taken seriously; suicide itself is all too common.

Intellectual difficulty, when it arises with confusion, poor explicit or narrative memory, or poor performance at work or studies, can be disheartening to an individual when they first become aware of it.

Failure at some tasks they previously were good at performing, for example, at solving crossword puzzles or routines at work, may lead them into depression secondary to the schizophrenic cognitive decline. They may find academic studies nearly impossible to fulfil, such as committing text to memory. This may be profoundly worrying to them because of its implications for their future employment and life's possibilities. Sometimes, after the initial shock of illness' onset, faculties may partially return, and with encouragement and perhaps their examinations being temporarily postponed by the authorities they may with perseverance be able to survive into tolerating their illness as only a very unpleasant aspect of their life.

Lack of interest and initiative and dulled emotion can be experienced by any schizophrenic patient but particularly those affected by negative symptoms. Inertia and lethargy may be experienced in the negative syndrome alongside tedium and stolidity, resulting in a complete absence of involvement with anyone or any activity. Patients with positive symptoms can also experience apathy, and this can lead to reluctance regarding self-care, which will require help to be reinstated. These symptoms arise from a total lack of experienced initiative or incentive, and need medication as well as enlivening social care to stimulate feelings of warmth, worthwhile effort and a connection with enjoyable aspects of life.

Pessimism and lack of hope may set in if the patient does not receive sufficient positive stimulation to offset the day-to-day realities of her illness. Even if the patient has been essentially lively and active, and she seems to be doing well in tolerating her condition with the help of medication, she may sink into pessimism nonetheless at any time; the contrast to her old familiar life, unpleasant as it may have been, can still feel too much for her to bear, and the effort required to keep going may be more than she can address, long term. Regular supportive outpatient Psychiatry appointments, or weekly supportive psychotherapy, may serve to maintain her interest in her life if she is already endeavouring to work with her hospital team.

Whether or not positive or negative symptoms are present, the patient may have a general awareness of unreality which may be uncomfortable to experience. This may become apparent to an observant clinician and may be helped if he addresses the non-psychotic part of her mind and sensitively pursues communication with her.

Personal isolation and withdrawal from others may in the long term create difficulties for the patient in the day-to-day management of her life. Lack of friends and contacts to help with food supplies or payment of bills, or social activities for shared enjoyment of human company may create a sad emptiness in the patient's life that she doesn't know how to fill. All the difficulties caused by her illness may cause shyness or reticence in approaching other people; she may require help to engage in a local community and may be either more or less willing to do so. Regular distractions such as weekly meetings in an art class or a walking group or a cookery session can create a sense of involvement with others, and also encourage self-help when doing the activities on her own.

The consciousness one infers from conversations with schizophrenic patients is that of the dissipation of meaningful experience, as seen in the sad young man at the start of this chapter. This consciousness is the idea of a baby in a pram abandoned for hours on end under a tree and consequently seeing only meaningless branches waving about against the sky, with no relief from a loving mum.

Esther Bick had the notion that a light nearby might stimulate a second, secure "skin" around the baby to contain its feelings and self:

> The need for a containing object would seem in the infantile unintegrated state to produce a frantic search for an object – a light, a voice, a smell, or other sensual object – which can hold the attention and thereby be experienced, momentarily at least, as holding the parts of the personality together.

> (Bick, 1968, p.484)
> (Reproduced with permission of The Harris Meltzer Trust)

For the adult schizophrenic patient, this light is a Psychoanalyst.

Schizophrenia is an illness that severely damages the patient's mind. If it starts in childhood the child's future is likely to be seriously adversely affected; treatment has not been found which can be preventive to the illness' limiting outcome. In adults, if effective treatment is not instigated immediately upon commencement of psychosis then the individual, commonly a young adult, will suffer an increasing "duration of untreated psychosis" and if not assisted therapeutically will slide into a mental state that is gradually destructive. When the patient's mind makes accommodation for the illness, her initiative, her intelligence, her personality, and her innate drive and outlook upon life will gradually fragment and crumble in response to the destruction, inertia, and despair caused by her schizophrenia.

If treatment can be begun immediately, ideally with interpretive, supportive, patient-centred psychoanalytic psychotherapy, the patient may be able to keep her mind intact as the young person she is, and will be able to discuss herself and her own perspective with a Psychiatry-trained Psychoanalyst. This is the most effective available therapy for schizophrenia. The prognosis with this treatment is potentially very good for a young person with enough energy and self-discipline to respond to it fully; her recovery may take years to effect but when she does find her mental health it will be very well based, and long-lasting. This treatment, assisted by medication, accesses the patient's unconscious mind, where her emotions are located, deep in the phylogenetically ancient limbic system of the brain, and eventually her brain's functioning as a whole will improve; her emotional life will have stabilised with her Psychoanalyst, and her brain's more recently developed cortical function of thinking, producing the manifest signs of psychosis, will not be disturbed by it. She will be surpassingly fortunate to receive this treatment, which at present is not available to all those who could benefit from it.

Nearly all other treatments for schizophrenia are palliative, leading to maintenance of the patient in her essentially compromised state. Some therapies, such as Need-Adapted treatment, may be successful in that the patient's functioning may be improved, an important aspect for her; but in most of them she will not have gained personal insight that would provide cure of her confusion. She will still struggle and feel unhappy if she has unanswered questions about herself. These are the limiting factors in her prognosis. Psychoanalytic psychotherapy allows all her questions to be answered by herself, her best source of understanding; her Psychoanalyst will have provided many answers and suggestions which have enabled her to do this. Much work is required to expand this treatment to all those who need it so badly.

References

Bick, E (1968). The experience of the skin in early object relations. p.484. *International Journal of Psychoanalysis,* 49: 484–6. Republished in The Tavistock Model: Collected Papers of Martha Harris and Esther Bick. Harris, M; Bick, E. Ed. Meg Harris Williams (2018), p.140. London: The Harris Meltzer Trust. Reproduced with permission of The Harris Meltzer Trust.

Crow, T (1980). Molecular pathology of schizophrenia: More than one disease process? *BMJ*, 280(6207): 66–8.

DSM-5-TR™ (2022). *Desk Reference to the Diagnostic Criteria from DSM-5-TR™*. American Psychiatric Association. Washington, DC: American Psychiatric Association Publishing.

Gelder, M; Harrison, P; Cowen, P (2006). *Shorter Oxford Textbook of Psychiatry*, 5th Edn. p.275. Oxford: Oxford University Press.

ICD-10 (1994). *Pocket Guide to the ICD-10 Classification of Mental and Behavioural Disorders*. World Health Organisation Geneva, Ed. Cooper, J. pp.93–4. USA and UK: Churchill Livingstone. Copyright Elsevier.

Lewis, Aubrey (1967). The psychopathology of insight. In: *Inquiries in Psychiatry: Clinical and Social Investigations*. 1st Edn. pp.16–29. London: Routledge and Kegan Paul. Reproduced by permission of Taylor and Francis Group.

Liddle, P (1987). The symptoms of chronic schizophrenia. A re-examination of the positive–negative dichotomy. *British Journal of Psychiatry*, **151**: 145–51.

Robbins, M (1993). *Experiences of Schizophrenia: An Integration of the Personal, Scientific and Therapeutic*. p.172. New York: Guilford Press.

Robbins, M (2012). The successful psychoanalytic therapy of a schizophrenic woman. pp.578–9. *Psychodynamic Psychiatry*, 40(4): 575–608. Reprinted with permission of Dr Michael Robbins and Guilford Press.

Psychoanalytic and psychotherapeutic approaches to schizophrenia

Chapter 4

The contribution of Psychoanalysis towards understanding schizophrenia

The classical psychoanalytic approach adopted since the days of Sigmund Freud himself has proved helpful to patients with a specific psychological disturbance due to unfortunate, emotionally disturbing, or incomprehensible experience earlier in their lives. They can work out for themselves their own understanding of themselves, from what their Psychoanalyst says to them. But schizophrenic patients cannot utilise classical psychoanalytical interpretations without the support of a psychotherapeutic approach because of the weakness of their ego and its vague boundaries. Psychotherapy is needed to support the patient; but the value of the interpretations of a psychoanalytical approach is that they stimulate change in the patient when she is stable enough to be able to respond to these communications of her Psychoanalyst. Psychoanalysis remains the theoretical root of psychoanalytic psychotherapy; yet while Psychiatry-trained Psychoanalysts who deliver the treatment select their own psychoanalytic approach to the mind from among the approaches developed by their forebears, each clinician initially needs fundamentally to adapt their theoretical approach into a patient-oriented technique which, equally, is tailored to each individual schizophrenic patient's needs. And Psychiatry training is required to recognise and manage psychosis in the clinical situation with a schizophrenic patient.

The application of Psychoanalysis to schizophrenia

Many Psychoanalysts since Freud's day have developed and amended his technique of Psychoanalysis for schizophrenic patients. Some of his followers founded separate schools of Psychoanalysis; the Kleinian

DOI: 10.4324/9781003433507-7

School in Britain, which developed object relations theory, is one example: it followed Melanie Klein's diversions from Freud; the American School of Ego Psychology was founded on Heinz Hartmann's and Edith Jacobson's ideas relating to aspects of Freud's structural theory. Some of these schools tried to help specifically schizophrenic patients; the Interpersonal-Relational School developed from the interpersonal approach of therapists and specialised in helping schizophrenic young men and women, again in America. Adherence to Freud's discipline of precisely timed psychoanalytic sessions is usually also accompanied, in the treatment of schizophrenic patients, by some intrusion of their mental disorganisation into an otherwise orderly therapeutic routine; they often need to be given psychoanalytic sessions in hospital.

The psychoanalytic concepts espoused by these schools adopt very broadly Freud's own original tenets. Psychiatry-trained Psychoanalysts adapt, in turn, their own psychoanalytic approach to their schizophrenic patients, in their own patient-centred technique, because this illness affects adversely and so fundamentally each mind's structure and nature in a way unique to each patient's personality. Each patient has their own personality, which has been affected by the illness with their own set of symptoms, even though the fact of psychosis is common to them all. Psychiatrists will have identified clinically the diagnosis of schizophrenia before treatment begins (see Chapter 3) so that the Psychiatry-trained Psychoanalyst knows the exact structure-type of his patient's mind and can tailor his work for the patient accordingly.

Schizophrenia is a discrete, identifiable illness although with a range of possible symptoms which therapy of the patient's mind resolves when successful. The overall aims of treatment can be summarised as follows:

i Initially, the patient's psychotic symptoms are quelled by antipsychotic medication.
ii The patient's personality needs become recognised and understood (by the Psychoanalyst, who then helps the patient) and resolved.
iii This leads eventually to affirmation of her more stable personality that will not produce psychotic symptoms.
iv The antipsychotic medication is reduced.

This medical aspect of psychological resolution of the illness, the aims of treatment, is a simplified perspective of the treatment process summarised by the four systems developed from Dr Robbins' Hierarchy of eight systems in his Theory of Mind, which identifies the functional levels of the patient as a whole human being at which therapy must intercede into the illness.

While medication is used to subdue brain malfunctioning when required, Psychoanalysis provides the basis for healing the patient's personal mental malfunctioning. In psychoanalytic psychotherapy, the psychoanalytic contribution is delivered as psychotherapy to provide much needed support for the patient. The psychoanalytic theories containing the perceptions of Freud and his followers, the forebears of today's Psychoanalytic Psychotherapists, may be seen to provide the rich basis from which contemporary clinicians can select their own technique. Often a historical clinician will have made specific observations from which they then developed their theories. Today's clinician can recognise some of these features in his schizophrenic patient. He may observe that his patient does not manifest either warmth or alternatively hostile feelings upon appropriate stimulation or events in her life; if he is familiar with Wilfred Bion's writing he will see for himself that his patient is destroying her own links to the rest of the world, of love and hate, through withdrawal from it. If his patient seems to oscillate between being mild and compliant some days, and aggressive attacks the next, he may observe clearly that her mind is in Klein's paranoid-schizoid position. It is quite possible for the clinician to be eclectic between psychoanalytic theories. Today's clinicians may even prefer to keep an open mind himself regarding which psychoanalytic phenomena his patient manifests, and treat her from a patient-centred perspective, remaining concerned always to relate to her as her highly unpredictable schizophrenic self and allowing theory to take a temporarily subsidiary position to his understanding and recognition of her features as an individual. This patient-oriented method of treatment does enable the patient to feel very cared for, even in her state of illness, and is practised in Turku, Finland, in the Need-Adapted approach which is practised there.

Symptoms initially may obscure a schizophrenic patient's personality and usually must be the focus at the start of treatment by the clinician. Medications prescribed for her by her Psychiatrist on the ward can be extremely helpful, and often with comparatively few side-effects to distract her, in keeping at bay her tendency towards psychotic language and behaviour. She may take time to overcome her psychotic tendency; and her therapist will be keeping a careful eye on this, to send her back to the ward in a taxi if it breaks out during a session, and to attend her in hospital for sessions while she is unwell. During this phase of her treatment, her Psychoanalyst may find it helpful to observe in his patient his forebears' insights that they have committed to paper and published. Psychoanalytic meetings and discussions are also important on an ongoing basis, and being able to extend his knowledge through information gleaned from the psychoanalytic literature will help him persevere in his work even when he may not be able to understand his schizophrenic patient for considerable periods at a time.

The Psychiatric Psychoanalyst's perspective

The Psychoanalyst treating a schizophrenic patient will find himself or herself attending her at times on her hospital ward, in an office allocated for the purpose. Here he will observe features of her psychosis. He will have this opportunity of detecting her deepest needs, as well as consolidating his relationship with her. Richard Lucas, in his book "The Psychotic Wavelength" (Lucas, 2009), sets out his idea of communicating with the psychotic patient when she is clinically psychotic. His approach is of helping the patient to feel understood and to live with a psychotic disorder rather than aspiring to resolve it entirely; in advocating communication and good humour while she is psychotic he tries to soften the patient's distress at herself and her illness. The Psychiatry-trained Psychoanalyst will at these times recognise her psychiatric symptoms and the features of psychosis observed by his Psychoanalytic forebears. Each of these historical clinicians' interpretations of their own observations, written down in the psychoanalytic literature, could potentially explain a connection for the Psychoanalyst between aspects of his patient's history, her experiences, and her present behaviour. He might observe that she becomes psychotic whenever her attention moves on to a particular person known to her. She might be communicating by her psychosis and behaviour with her Psychoanalyst that during her experience of growing up her carers "drove her crazy", a process Harold Searles described. The Psychoanalyst may feel that his time spent with her in her psychotic state is being wasted, but it is very likely that, instead, she will be experiencing his presence with her through her transference to him, and taking encouragement and confirmation of her own validity and her identity from this.

As the schizophrenic patient progresses in her treatment, her psychotic tendency subsides due to her own increasing understanding of herself, which is due to her Psychoanalyst's understanding of her that he has communicated to her each week during her sessions. Once she has become more insightful and has become more like the person she was, perhaps, at the start of her life, before she began reacting to her environments (Hingley, 2006) as evidenced in her representational world (which her Psychoanalyst will have been able to identify in a general way from all he knows about her early life), her Psychoanalyst may revert to the psychoanalytic theory he studied and applied during his psychoanalytic training. By now, he will be beginning to understand her personality as an individual rather than regarding her as "a schizophrenic patient".

When his patient's tendency towards psychosis has subsided and she is able to talk with him in a cogent and comprehensible manner, the Psychoanalyst is likely to adhere to his Theory of Mind and the psychoanalytic principles he adopted during his training so that he can frame his view of how to proceed with his patient's treatment. Dr Michael Robbins stated clearly that he adhered to no specific school of Psychoanalysis. Dr Leslie Sohn treated schizoaffective patients with a Kleinian approach, espousing object relations theory and recognising projective identification in them; in addition, he maintained that it is necessary when treating a schizophrenic patient to do a mental state examination "every 5 minutes" in order to detect any element of psychosis before it generalises and the patient becomes ill during a session away from hospital. In this event, the patient should be sent back to the hospital in a taxi and be visited by her Psychoanalyst when he is able to see her there.

The Psychiatry-trained Psychoanalyst treating a schizophrenic patient will hope to see her personality begin to emerge once her psychotic symptoms have not only been controlled by medication but have also been addressed at their sources. He will be glad to find his patient recovered to this extent and now will aim to strengthen her in her abilities to perceive realistically, develop her autonomy, and defend herself effectively in her relations with other people, including her family when she interacts with them. She herself will be enhancing her awareness after years of confinement by her developing and then manifest illness. She will be relieved to be able to think clearly after a long period of confusion, and to reject ideas that she may have grown up with in her family but, not understanding any alternative, will have been living with despite her better judgement. Now that she understands what she thinks and has for a long time been trying to identify, she feels much happier; and this allows her to function normally, with little in her mind that would be likely ever to create psychosis in her again, even on reduced medication. Her healing has come about through her Psychoanalyst's professional relationship with her, his approbation of the medication she has been receiving, and her own responses to her Psychoanalyst and to her medication. The role of Psychoanalysis in her healing has been the discipline of her attending her sessions and her Psychoanalyst's psychoanalytic understanding of schizophrenia presented by his psychoanalytic antecedents and, perhaps, also some more recent psychoanalytic frameworks suggested for treating the illness (Dr Robbins' seven therapeutic Stages, the Hierarchy of four of his Systems, and the PPCC theory; see Chapter 7).

Each Psychiatry-trained Psychoanalyst of schizophrenic and schizoaffective patients addresses first the patient's symptoms; then he endeavours to understand his patient as a person, familiarising himself with her personality and its tendencies, any assumptions she might be making that require adjustment, her grasp of reality and of issues that ought to be more aligned with her own circumstances and situations, and of difficulties that she might be experiencing which he could help her with by discussing possibilities with her. He will see her as a discrete individual in this way, but will also understand her mind through his chosen Psychoanalytic school within which he trained. The patient's psychosis has abated, partly through use of medication and partly through the Psychoanalyst substantively alleviating the unconscious factors which provoked it, by identifying these and interpreting and rendering them innocuous, "chimney-sweeping", through Breuer's patient Anna O's "talking cure" technique (Quinodoz, 2004). The Psychoanalyst can now concentrate on developing his patient's wellbeing and abilities in functioning with other people, socially engaging in activities which she might have already been able to start herself, in hospital or in her own community. He will discuss the issues she raises with him and confirm in her strengths that she is developing.

During periods of time when the Psychoanalyst is uncertain about what is happening with his patient's mind when she is not overtly psychotic, he will return to his understanding of how the human mind behaves, derived from one or more Psychoanalytic clinician-writers of the past, together with discussions and meetings from his training at his Institute. It is from these sources, too, that he will have been able to learn specifically about how these authors understood schizophrenia. The two fundamental psychological aspects of schizophrenia as it affects patients, thus its symptoms, and the nature of the personalities of ex-schizophrenia sufferers, are quite different from each other. To date, there are not enough recovered schizophrenic patients to know how their personalities differ from non-schizophrenic individuals. They may be as varied as in the healthy population. Anti-psychotic medications only affect psychotic symptoms. While the patient is potentially psychotic, the Psychoanalyst principally tries carefully to address symptomatic aspects of what he detects in her; he will be keeping in mind her nascent personality behind her symptoms and working in a patient-centred way with humanity and common sense to try to alleviate her suffering. At this time, he will have in mind, as already noted, the understanding of his Psychoanalytic forebears on the phenomena manifest in his own observations of his patient. These clinicians, particularly Bion, offered their theories on the schizophrenic process; as described above, Bion thought that schizophrenic patients destroy their own "links of love, hate and knowledge" (Bion, 1962, pp.42–9) and, as noted, this might be helpful to the Psychoanalyst in recognising this happening when his own patient fails to respond to him or remains otherwise disengaged when a warm response might have been expected.

When a schizophrenic patient is potentially psychotic her Psychoanalyst depends both on his own intuition and clinical skills and finds useful the work of his forebears on schizophrenic symptoms and characteristics; when she is no longer likely to become psychotic he may find psychoanalytic literature, in general, a good guide to follow in treating her, perhaps having chosen one school in preference over others. There is a stage when there is no sharp distinction between these two different phases, even though they differ from each other; the early one merges into the second, and the sequence (i)–(iv) outlined above proceeds as a continuum. The details of the process are described in Chapter 7.

Patient safety is a priority at all times, from the very start of treatment to its outcome. Schizophrenic patients are unpredictable, particularly at the start of treatment and as it proceeds, while the patient's personality becomes established and understood by the Psychoanalyst and also by the staff at the hospital where she is accommodated, until she acquires this. Loyalty is a strong force that can be utilised in the service of patient safety. Even during the early days while the patient is potentially psychotic, her loyalty to the staff on her hospital ward acts as a strong influence towards keeping her safe while travelling to her Psychoanalyst's consulting room. Her Psychoanalyst's skill keeps her psychosis at bay while he gently engages her in dialogue. Emotions will be aroused, but she will be trying to cooperate with him and with the ward staff, and her attachments to both are everyone's greatest investment. The collective experience of understanding schizophrenia and treating it, which helps the Psychoanalyst and the ward staff alike to care for the patient, is made all the more effective through the patient's loyalty to them.

Influential Psychoanalysts

Many Psychoanalysts have in the past observed the illness "schizophrenia", and Neuropsychoanalysts have tried to understand their observations, in terms of both the schizophrenic individual as a patient and her brain as the highly complex organ that largely, together with systemic emotions and environmental experiences, determines her mind. Their writings have interested and inspired subsequent generations of clinicians, both Psychiatrists and Psychoanalysts, and particularly those clinicians qualified in both approaches, to treat, try to understand further, and eventually to resolve the illness. Observations that are widely replicated are especially useful for understanding their implications in schizophrenic patients generally. In considering these characteristics of schizophrenia, working at understanding them, and then writing about them, these clinicians assist future clinicians to help future patients. Discussing the findings helps to establish facts about the illness upon which today's Psychiatry-trained Psychoanalyst may gratefully depend as he encounters his own patients, when they initially may present to him a very confusing picture. Some past Psychoanalysts produced particularly substantive and helpful work in this endeavour.

Sigmund Freud

Freud, early in his studies, pointed out the narcissism of the schizophrenic patient, i.e. the turning inwards of the patient and loss of all participation in the external world. He linked this to the patient's lack of libido, or energy source, and sexualised the origin of the illness. Not many clinicians today would necessarily agree with the sexualisation of the illness, but observation of schizophrenic patients does almost universally reveal their lack of outside interests and of any inclination to explore the world.

Freud tried to understand schizophrenic patients' use of language rather than trying to develop and utilise a transference with them. He considered that, for a schizophrenic patient, a word carries the value of the object most people feel it merely describes; he also observed that schizophrenic patients treat concrete things as though they were abstract like the words that describe them. This confusion between the concrete and the abstract was again noted by Hanna Segal (see below). Freud observed that schizophrenic patients do not make connection between word-cathexes (in their preconscious) and thing-cathexes (in their unconscious), i.e. between the meanings of a word and the thing it describes; the relationship between the meanings of words and things is absent, leaving only confusion. For these patients, the cathexis of their unconscious mind is withdrawn, and their mind seems to function largely at a teleological level.

Freud was very pleased that the Psychiatrist Eugen Bleuler acknowledged in his book of 1911 (Bleuler, 1911) the contribution Psychoanalysis might make to understanding schizophrenia. But Bleuler eventually rejected Psychoanalysis and resigned from his membership of the International Psycho-Analytical Association. However, Freud writes in "An Autobiographical Study" (Freud, 1925) that "Bleuler, in 1906, demonstrated the existence in various psychoses of mechanisms like those which analysis had discovered in neurotics". Freud goes on to write: "Since then analysts have never relaxed their efforts to come to an understanding of the psychoses". All the Psychoanalysts since Freud who have studied schizophrenia in patients have justified this statement by Freud in 1925.

Melanie Klein

Melanie Klein was one of the first to disagree with Freud in his view that schizophrenic patients could not develop a transference and so could not be analysed. Klein showed that both positive and negative transferences could be developed with these patients, and moreover that a Psychoanalyst cannot analyse one without the other; and Freud changed his opinion.

Klein observed that schizophrenic patients are very well defended, adopting particularly splitting and projective identification as means they commonly use to defend themselves against anxieties. In the paranoid-schizoid position, a concept that she developed with Ronald

Fairbairn where the individual considers separately the good and bad aspects of another person, there is an unresolved tendency towards splitting (separating off from the self an unwanted part, often bad but sometimes good) and projective identification (sending parts of the self into another person with whom the subject now identifies). There is only a weak capacity to integrate the split-off parts of the ego. The individual has a greater tendency to split in order to avoid anxiety aroused by the destructive impulses directed against the self and external world; this can lead to a state of fragmentation, and also makes it impossible to work through the early anxieties.

Klein's view is that these processes underlie the schizophrenic patient's experiences, particularly of loneliness, and also of confusion which she attributes particularly to fragmentation of the ego and the excessive use of projective identification. The schizophrenic patient can neither understand nor trust herself. She wishes to make relationships with other people but cannot. However, Klein believes, "as a fact", as she has written, that even schizophrenic patients have an urge towards integration and have a relation, however undeveloped, to the good object and the good self.

Splitting mechanisms allow the ego to defend itself against persecutory anxiety, and form the basis of the dissociated and disintegrated condition of the schizophrenic patient. Klein contrasts persecutory with depressive anxiety and clarifies that schizophrenia, mania, and depression could combine, as in schizoaffective disorder, due to interaction by both development and regression between the infantile paranoid-schizoid and depressive positions.

Schizophrenic dissociation seems to Klein to be a regression to infantile states of disintegration. For the infant, gratification by the external good object again and again helps to break through schizoid states of disintegration due to splitting; but the adult schizophrenic patient's mind is not so elastic, and she is not helped by her maternal good object in the same way as the child.

Schizoid defences are often manifest in schizophrenic patients. These patients sometimes maintain a passive rejection of the Psychoanalyst's interpretations (see Stage 1 of Dr Michael Robbins' seven stages of psychoanalytic psychotherapy in Chapter 7) through lack of emotional engagement with him accompanied by an absence of the usual basic level of helpful curiosity. The patient's flat affect may obscure a potential transference, which the perceptive Psychoanalyst will have detected before accepting her as his patient. Splitting off from herself of impulses felt to be dangerous and hostile, and directing these at her Psychoanalyst in projective identification, keep her paranoid anxiety in a latent state. She may, alternatively, turn her destructive impulses towards her own ego, so that parts of her ego temporarily go out of existence. The relief of anxiety can permit introjection of the Psychoanalyst as a good object, thereby allowing strengthening and integration of her ego. Psychoanalytic processes aim to help her to diminish splitting and projective identification and come nearer to experiencing the depressive position.

Guilt and depressive anxiety in a patient refer to that part of the ego which is felt to contain the good object and therefore to be the good part; the patient's guilt in the depressive position (Klein, 1935) arises from her destroying something good in herself, possibly due to having damaged her good object. In the schizophrenic patient, owing to processes of fragmentation, she weakens her ego through splitting part of it away; depressive anxiety and guilt are very strongly split off. The parts of the schizophrenic patient's mind, in the paranoid-schizoid position (Klein, 1946), that experience guilt and depressive anxiety are felt to be out of reach by the patient, Klein thinks, and so are difficult to access in the analysis.

In schizophrenic patients, Klein thinks the super-ego becomes al-most indistinguishable from their destructive impulses and internal persecutors. She feels that such an overwhelming super-ego, an agency often tyrannical in the infantile mind as she demonstrated in her work with children, plays an important part in schizophrenia. Klein's view is that the early super-ego, built up when oral-sadistic impulses and phantasies are at their height, underlies psychosis; oral-sadism has a very important role in schizophrenia. There is an early stage of mental development at which sadism becomes active at all the various sources of libidinal pleasure. Klein observes that the Oedipus conflict begins at a period when sadism predominates, i.e. the first three months of life, corresponding to the early phase of the paranoid-schizoid position. Melanie Klein identifies (Klein, 1946) the persecutory anxieties of the paranoid-schizoid position as providing the fixation-point for schizophrenic illness in adult life.

Klein observes that a severe inhibition of the capacity to form and use symbols, and so to develop phantasy life, and the resulting disturbance in the relation to the external world and to reality are characteristic of schizophrenia. Hanna Segal made her own observations of this phenomenon (see below).

Klein also found that interpretations of schizoid states are challenging to our capacity to put the interpretations to the patient in an intellectually clear form in which the links between the conscious, pre-conscious, and unconscious are established. She thinks that this is especially important when only the intellect of the patient is available and not her emotions, which is usually the case with schizophrenic patients, especially near the start of treatment. And, like Freud, she expresses hopes for the continued development of the Psychoanalysis of schizophrenic patients in future work.

Wilfred Bion

Wilfred Bion expresses his view in his book "Second Thoughts" (1967) that the Psychoanalysis of a schizophrenic is done with the patient alone or not at all. He considers that the illness is so complex that any outside interference with the analytic process would distort it. He concurs with Klein, from whom he learnt as a student, that projective identification, where the patient's own ill feelings can be felt by another person, frequently occurs in schizophrenic patients. He also considers that schizophrenic patients fracture their loving relations with other people; they cancel and no longer feel emotions such as hatred or continue interests they may have earlier experienced. Terminating these links of love, hate, and knowledge occurs as the patient withdraws into herself with the progression of the illness. Schizophrenic patients' own perceptive apparatus is destroyed by themselves, with a consequent mental state that is neither alive nor dead.

Bion maintains that projective identification of conscious awareness and the associated "inchoation [beginnings, birth] of verbal thought" is central to the differentiation of the psychotic from the non-psychotic personality. He believes this starts right at the beginning of the patient's life with a developing gap between the psychotic and the non-psychotic that cannot be bridged by the patient. Bion argues that these sadistic attacks on the ego and on the foundations of inchoate (nascent) verbal thought, together with the projective identification of the fragments, ensures that from this point on there is an ever-widening divergence between the psychotic and the non-psychotic parts of the personality, so that eventually the gulf is felt to be unbridgeable.

This gulf is clearly illustrated by the schism between the two parts, psychotic (Determining Orientation) and non-psychotic (Observations), in the diagram for schizophrenia in the PPCC model of the schizophrenic patient's mind as it progresses from illness to health and integration (see Figures 7.2 and 7.4).

Bion was greatly influenced by Melanie Klein. He agreed with her observations in schizophrenic patients of splitting and projective identification, and that these can be helped to resolve; he believed that if splitting has been adequately worked through the tendency to split the object and the ego at the same time is restrained. Each session can then proceed towards ego development.

Bion considers that the patient may feel a failure, imprisoned in her state of mind, and subjected to attack by expelled particles of ego that lead to an independent and uncontrolled existence outside her personality. These particles contain or are contained by external objects and are hostile to the patient, who feels surrounded by bizarre objects. Real objects such as Bion's example of a gramophone are surrounded by pieces of the patient's personality, for example, the part that sees or the part that hears; and these particles become responsive, e.g. they can watch or listen, depending on the piece of personality surrounding them; the gramophone may then be felt to be watching or listening to the patient. The particles are used as ideas and later words by the patient so that words are felt by her to be the actual things they name; confusions then arise because the patient equates but does not symbolise (see Hanna Segal below).

Bion's view of the schizophrenic patient's transference with the Psychoanalyst is that it is premature, precipitate, and intensely dependent. Under pressure from her life or death instincts, projective identification with the Psychoanalyst as object becomes overactive, leading to painful confusional states. Whichever of the life or death instincts is dominant tries to express itself through mental activities which, however, are subjected to mutilation by the other, temporarily subordinated instinct. Endeavouring to avoid the confusional states and injured by the mutilations, the patient tries to restore the transference relationship, even though it is quite featureless. This combination of characteristics leads to massive utilisation of projective identification.

Bion considers, like Melanie Klein, that at the onset of the infantile depressive position, elements of verbal thought increase in intensity and depth. In consequence, the pains of psychic reality are exacerbated by it; the patient who regresses to the paranoid-schizoid position, as does she who develops a schizophrenic illness, will, as she does so, turn destructively on her embryonic capacity for verbal thought as one of the elements which have led to her pain.

These thoughts of Bion about schizophrenic verbal symptom development, like the thoughts of Freud about word handling by schizophrenic patients, are cogent and psychologically explanatory. At the present time, we do not know details about how the prefrontal cortex, which processes words and actions in the brain, develops shortly after birth, at the time when words begin to be formed by the infant. The baby's mind and its brain develop together; and at present, as Bion has done, following an observable train of development with cogent theory is the best guide we have towards understanding later psychological illnesses' origins and manifestations, albeit arising from a physiological basis which is not as yet understood.

More clinically, the Psychoanalyst will bear these considerations in mind as he relates to his patient's struggles with her confusion and her feelings as affected by her illness symptoms. Even if a schizophrenic patient achieves a realisation of psychic reality viz. she realises she has hallucinations and delusions, she may deeply resent the Psychoanalyst and bear him powerful feelings of hatred. She may be quite aware that she is insane, stating this clearly, but blame the Psychoanalyst for this. She may calm down and declare she feels better, but the analytic work must continue, so that the changes in her object relationships brought about by her recognition of her insanity can be investigated in detail.

Bion emphasises the damage to the analysis that will be done if the Psychoanalyst attempts to reassure the patient and so undoes all the good work that has led to her being able to realise the severity of her condition. The Psychoanalyst has created with the patient an opportunity, which must not be lost, for exploring with the patient "what it means to do analytic or any other kind of work when insane".

Hanna Segal

Hanna Segal, also a student of Klein, thought that the psychotic individual regresses to very early infancy, a phase of development that manifests elements of the illness. She believed that within aspects of very early life could be detected factors which indicate future problems for the individual's health. Hanna Segal identified the phenomenon of "symbolic equation", whereby a schizophrenic patient mistakes a symbol for the thing it represents; she equates the object with its symbol (Segal, 1981). This conflation relates to Freud's observation that, in schizophrenic patients, a word may become a thing in itself. Segal relates that through her work with a schizophrenic patient, Edward, he was able to live through 20 years of useful life, marrying, having a family, and working professionally. She demonstrated, like Klein's and Bion's successes, that schizophrenia is amenable to psychoanalytic intervention, even if further support for the patient is also required at times.

Herbert Rosenfeld

Herbert Rosenfeld, another of Klein's students, also worked with schizophrenic patients, and was particularly interested in the narcissism apparent in them, i.e. their tendency to turn inwards and suffer omnipotent object relations which is a defence against envy and dependence; to deal with her envy the patient devalues her objects. He reinforced the view, held by Klein and Bion, that projective identification features significantly within the schizophrenic patient's mind. Rosenfeld treated a schizoid patient he called Mildred entirely with Psychoanalysis, which at the time was not thought possible.

Anna Freud

Anna Freud, the daughter of Sigmund Freud, energetically defended her father's work from all adjustment by others, particularly from Melanie Klein's divergent professional views during the Controversial Discussions of 1941 (King et al., 1991). She was, herself, especially interested in the health and wellbeing of children, and the Anna Freud Centre for Child Health, previously the Hampstead Clinic, was established in her honour. She did not express many views about schizophrenia as it affects children, but preserved her father's legacy about it.

Joseph Sandler

Joseph Sandler, a student of Anna Freud who worked with her at the Hampstead Clinic, developed useful concepts relating to his interest in child Psychoanalysis, such as the need for a background of safety, much used by later Psychoanalysts. His representational world, conceived of together with Bernard Rosenblatt (Sandler et al., 1962), is fundamental to the PPCC theory of the psychoanalytic process by which schizophrenia may be resolved and thereby provides a connection between understanding schizophrenia and psychoanalytic theory. The representational world is the representation in a child's or an adult's mind of an accumulation of significant features of the environments they have lived in, to date; this representation is amended as the child grows up or as the adult becomes well in treatment and is useful both to the child, unconsciously, as a guide in future environments, and to the Psychoanalyst while he sees his schizophrenic patient's impression of her past life becoming more positively amended as her health improves.

Frieda Fromm-Reichmann

Frieda Fromm-Reichmann treated schizophrenic patients at Chestnut Lodge in Maryland, USA, with an interpersonal-relational approach that became, with other members, the Interpersonal School in the 1940s and 1950s. She was entirely compassionate towards her patients and talked with them about their experiences in a rational and sympathetic manner. The approach that considers the patient as an individual to whom the clinician is relating has benefited psychoanalytic thinking, and the Interpersonal School forged close links with the Object Relations Schools, in particular (Greenberg et al., 1983).

Harry Stack Sullivan

Harry Stack Sullivan developed Interpersonal Psychiatry, though he never tried to become a Psychoanalyst. He was a contributor to the interpersonal-relational approach, rejecting Freud's adherence to intrapsychic mechanisms as an explanation for human behaviour, and he saw them as obscuring a person's problems by assuming a spurious divide between the person and his environment. He believed that schizophrenia is an understandable reaction to interpersonal anxiety; this anxiety, which starts very early in life, is so overwhelming that it instigates and promotes the dissociative component of the personality.

Richard Lucas

Richard Lucas, a Psychiatrist and Psychoanalyst, was of the view that it is possible to communicate "on the psychotic wavelength" with the schizophrenic patient while she is psychotic (Lucas, 2009). He maintains that if this is done it is comforting to the patient because it allows contact with an otherwise apparently inaccessible part of her mind. Rational, non-psychotic communication remains the principal means of communicating with her, but some useful understanding may nonetheless be gained from spending time with her when she is psychotic.

Brian Martindale and Alison Summers

Brian Martindale and Alison Summers together developed a useful understanding of how psychodynamic thinking can elucidate psychotic phenomena (Martindale et al., 2013). By considering the symbolic content of language uttered by a psychotic patient its meaning in reality may sometimes be uncovered. Once its meaning has been deciphered, the patient may be helped in practice, where she has experienced her problem. Her psychotic defence will have been the best language her brain could produce to try to explain to the clinician what her problem is, or what her injured feelings consist of. Psychodynamics may be utilised to unravel psychotic language and is particularly useful in early intervention interviews with a young person who is experiencing her first psychotic breakdown. Here the experienced clinician may be able to recognise through psychodynamics the meanings underlying the young person's distress, and so be able to resolve them for her, more than simple recognition of her psychosis as such could achieve.

Elvin Semrad

Elvin Semrad was Dr Michael Robbins' mentor at the Massachusetts Mental Health Center. He taught Dr Robbins how to sit with his schizophrenic patients while they experienced, tolerated, and worked through the terrible feelings resulting from their life's experiences before they arrived at his consulting-room, to find him ready and willing to help them through their ordeal. The Psychoanalyst has to be able to tolerate the feelings that his patient has; in his case it is by proxy, but this can still be difficult for him. Elvin Semrad showed Dr Robbins that it can be done and is necessary in order to be able to help the patient to do this herself, and then to move on to better ways of relating to and experiencing life.

Michael Robbins

The Psychiatrist and Psychoanalyst Michael Robbins is frequently mentioned in this text. In particular, his clinical technique, his written accounts, his identification of the seven stages of his therapeutic technique, and four therapeutically accessible Systems of the Hierarchy he proposes which can achieve resolution of schizophrenia in his patients, provide a firm basis for further Psychoanalysts to explore for themselves the kind of work he has produced (Robbins, 1993, 2012).

The British Psychoanalytical Society and the Institute of Psycho-Analysis

The British Psychoanalytical Society, formed on 20 February 1919, and the Institute of Psycho-Analysis, set up in 1924, became divided after the Controversial Discussions of 1941 which had developed mainly because Anna Freud could not accept the veracity of Melanie Klein's clinical divergence from her own father, Sigmund Freud's, theories. A compromise was reached, generally known as the "Gentlemen's Agreement", whereby there would be three groups of Psychoanalysts, those following Melanie Klein's theory and technique in the Kleinian School, those following Anna Freud and Sigmund Freud in the Viennese or 'B' group, and the Middle Group of "Independents" who really were eclectic and maintained their right to learn from all reasonable sources of knowledge.

In Britain, most Psychoanalysts today choose to train in the Kleinian School, but there are members practising in all three schools. Klein's, Bion's, Segal's, and Rosenfeld's ideas are all consistent and adhered to within the Kleinian School. Anna Freud's and Joseph Sandler's work at the Hampstead Clinic, now the Anna Freud Centre, concentrates on child health and teaches many Psychoanalysts and clinicians concerned with child welfare. Independent Psychoanalysts relate to each other with their own models. Today's Psychoanalysts, if they train in the Kleinian School, may understand and adopt the teachings of Klein, Bion, Segal, and Rosenfeld together, since these are all compatible with each other, based as they are on Klein's object relations approach. This is the largest body of psychoanalytic understanding about schizophrenic illness, which the Psychoanalytic trainee may find more supportive to him in his learning than any other source. It engages with child Psychoanalysis; but the Anna Freud Centre also does a great deal of successful work with children and their families. The British Psychoanalytical Society offers its Members "a wide range of approaches to psychoanalysis compared with what is offered in many Societies and Institutes in the International Psychoanalytical Association" (King et al., 1991).

References

Bion, W (1962). *Learning from Experience*. pp.42–9. London: Karnac.

Bion, W (1967). *Second Thoughts*. London, New York: Karnac.

Bleuler, E (1911). *Dementia Praecox, or the Group of Schizophrenias*. Tr. New York, 1950.

Freud, S (1925). An autobiographical study. In: *The Standard Edition of the Complete Psychological Works of Sigmund Freud*, Ed. Strachey, J. Vol. XX, p.61. London: Vintage (2001).

Greenberg, J; Mitchell, S (1983). *Object Relations in Psychoanalytic Theory*. Cambridge, MA: Harvard University Press.

Hingley, S (2006). Finding meaning within psychosis: The contribution of psychodynamic theory and practice. In: *Evolving Psychosis: Different Stages, Different Treatments*. Eds. Johannessen, J; Martindale, B; Cullberg, J. pp. 200–214. London and New York: Routledge.

King, P; Steiner, R, Eds. (1991). *The Freud-Klein Controversies 1941–45*. London: Routledge.

Klein, M (1935). A contribution to the psychogenesis of manic-depressive states. In: *Love, Guilt and Reparation and Other Works 1921–1945*. Ed. Hanna Segal, pp. 262–289. London: Vintage, 1998.

Klein, M (1946). Notes on some schizoid mechanisms. In: *Envy and Gratitude and Other Works 1946–1963*. Eds. Masud, M; Khan, R. pp. 1–24. London: Hogarth Press, 1984.

Lucas, R (2009). *The Psychotic Wavelength*. London and New York: Routledge.

Martindale, B; Summers, A (2013). The psychodynamics of psychosis. *Advances in Psychiatric Treatment*, 19: 124–31.

Quinodoz, J-M (2004). *Reading Freud: A Chronological Exploration of Freud's Writings*. London and New York: Routledge.

Robbins, M (1993). *Experiences of Schizophrenia: An Integration of the Personal, Scientific, and Therapeutic*. New York: Guilford Press.

Robbins, M (2012). The successful psychoanalytic therapy of a schizophrenic woman. *Psychodynamic Psychiatry*, 40(4): 575–608.

Sandler, J; Rosenblatt, B (1962). The concept of the representational world. *Psychoanalytic Study of the Child*, 17: 128–45.

Segal, H (1981). *Delusion and Artistic Creativity & Other Psychoanalytic Essays. The Work of Hanna Segal*. London: Free Association Books.

Chapter 5

Psychoanalytic and non-psychoanalytic features of psychoanalytic psychotherapy for schizophrenia

The practice of psychoanalytic psychotherapy employs several different aspects of Sigmund Freud's technique of Psychoanalysis. Freud's original, classical approach is traditionally very strict in its stipulations of the conduct of the therapy, its parameters, and its management of such aspects as time and its financing. All Freud's contemporaries followed these guidelines laid down by him. But classical Psychoanalysis is infrequently practised today. More common is therapy based upon psychoanalytic principles that diverge from it in some way, often in the direction of providing support for the patient in the manner of psychotherapy; this allows the patient to receive interpretations which can intercede helpfully into her mind, thus informing her about herself, while at the same time strengthening her handling of the therapy and of her life. Psychotherapeutic, supportive therapy is the therapeutic medium through which the incisive, interpretive, curative, and psychoanalytic elements of the treatment are delivered to the patient, in a form she can absorb and utilise. Psychoanalytic psychotherapy of schizophrenic patients adopts several aspects of classical Psychoanalysis as its framework, whichever School of Psychoanalysis is adhered to by the Psychoanalyst, while maintaining a supportive psychotherapeutic approach to the treatment.

Psychoanalytic features

Psychoanalytic psychotherapy is today gaining recognition as one of the most helpful and successful approaches towards resolving mental illnesses of different kinds, as well as sustaining essentially well people who require support when they are especially stressed and strained. Jonathan Shedler (2010) and others have demonstrated through research

DOI: 10.4324/9781003433507-8

the greater efficacy of psychodynamic psychotherapy, which is similar to psychoanalytic psychotherapy in addressing the patient's unconscious mind, over other techniques numerically, in terms of statistical effect sizes. Shedler points out that some therapeutic techniques such as cognitive behavioural therapy (CBT) even "borrow" aspects of psychodynamic psychotherapy without acknowledging this. The unconscious part of the mind, which interested Sigmund Freud although he maintained that he did not discover it but rather discovered the way to examine and understand it, houses much of the disturbance manifest in mental illnesses. Freud recognised that neurotic patients repress down into the unconscious those elements of mental life that the mind rejects, for a number of different reasons, and that psychotic patients project outwards these elements into others, in order to protect themselves from them.

The unconscious mind of schizophrenic patients is very disturbed indeed. It engages in Freud's conception of "primary process" activities, i.e. according to him, "the free and uninhibited flow of psychic energy", which is not organised and can harbour traumatic memories that can burst through into the patient's conscious mind as psychosis. The concept of the unconscious mind is helpful to psychodynamic psychotherapists and to all Psychoanalysts, including those psychoanalysing schizophrenic patients, since it accommodates the substance of the patient's trauma; it is distinguished from the cogent, logical language even the confused schizophrenic patient uses sometimes in conversation with him, the Psychoanalyst. Dr Michael Robbins has greatly developed understanding of psychoanalytic psychotherapy for schizophrenic patients (Robbins, 1993). The PPCC model (Steggles, 2019) supports Dr Robbins' work and indicates clearly the division in schizophrenia between the patient's conscious thoughts or observations and the psychotic illness they suffer, at the Observations and Determining Orientation variables, respectively (see Figure 7.4). The Internal Space of the PPCC model represents affect regulation and all the other functions that take place in the unconscious mind; when the unconscious is very disturbed, as in the schizophrenic patient, affect regulation and other functions become dysregulated, adding to the confusion of the patient's psychotic state.

The transference of a patient is the transference of her feelings from people or objects she knows onto her Psychoanalyst in the therapeutic situation. It is one of the main indicators for the Psychoanalyst that an individual would be likely to respond to his interpretations if she became his patient. Selection of schizophrenic patients is very important before therapy is commenced, because the illness can damage irrecoverably a patient's mind and render therapeutic success unlikely. Also, the process of recovery with psychoanalytic psychotherapy can make such great demands upon the patient that she may feel she cannot continue with it; this would be a disappointment to her, to her Psychoanalyst, and to others who have invested in her treatment. The transference, however, can show the Psychoanalyst to what extent she is likely to be able to respond to him, even when she feels negative emotions or does not understand her situations during treatment. A strong transference augurs well for the patient's adherence to her treatment.

Freud emphasised the general importance of a patient's transference, and it became a consistent feature of his first psychoanalytic cases. Early on in his psychoanalytic evaluation of schizophrenic patients, however, he did not feel they could develop a transference at all. Later, though, he changed his view, and agreed with Melanie Klein that they could indeed be analysed using their transference; she had discovered that both positive and negative transferences could develop, and that both needed to be analysed rather than one only. Freud's main clinical encounter with a schizophrenic patient was with Judge Schreber (Freud, 1911), but this was a complex case whose symptom details greatly interested Freud, and he did not study specifically Judge Schreber's transference onto him except to write that the Judge transferred onto Freud the feelings he had had for his father and his brother before their deaths.

The main technique Freud adopted in his new psychoanalytic treatment for resolving his patients' difficulties was that he would persuade them to talk freely for a while, i.e. freely associate, and then he would interpret what they had just said in terms of the background to their condition, the other verbal contents they had offered to him, and his own thoughts on what might be the cause of their problems. Interpretations thus make considerable inroads into the patient's mind, her life, and explorations into her presenting difficulty. They should be made kindly and with tact, since the patient has to accept them and absorb them; if they are palatable to her she is much more likely to be able to do this. They should always be accurate and correct according to the Psychoanalyst's best analytic deductions, and never pejorative or dismissive. He should frame them helpfully, which assists the transference and the progress of the analysis, and should be aimed at elucidating for the patient the most likely explanations for her feelings, her behaviour, and for the nature of her experiences given, for example, certain preceding events which might have coloured these in a particular way.

Enlightening the patient about herself in this way is an excellent method of helping her to understand herself when previously she has really been in the dark regarding many aspects of her life. The more she understands about herself in a kindly light the happier she will become, and the better able she is to engage in activities which require her to use her mind for everyone's benefit and especially her own, at work, in recreation, or in her family life. A correct interpretation puts the Psychoanalyst's finger on exactly what the psychological reason has been for a problem mystifying her, and she feels great relief as if from a heavy weight which had been preventing her from functioning properly. Often these problems are difficulties in her unconscious, which she certainly could not have worked out on her own. Interpretations are the instrument which tackles specifically the unconscious roots of the patient's mental, emotional, or behavioural vagaries which have concerned her, which brought her to her Psychoanalyst's door. Through bringing these root causes into her conscious mind her Psychoanalyst achieves relief for her mind's tension and distress, and shows her consciously the measures she might take in her mental approach or her arrangements to avoid continuation of her problematic circumstance. Once she understands her mind's problematic tendencies, she can do something about preventing them from having their effects in the future; he shows her how to avoid her illness.

Even if the patient's illness is as serious as schizophrenia or schizoaffective disorder, the Psychoanalyst's interventions will be heard in the context of the sound of his voice and in his comforting presence. To start with, early in treatment, he will not make direct interpretations to the patient. He is much more likely to engage fully in establishing rapport with her, expressing kindly and sympathetically what he can understand about her pain and predicament, and building the therapeutic alliance (Zetzel, 1970). Once she has stabilised in his care he may comment upon aspects of what she has said, as suggestions to her, stimulating her to agree or to disagree with him. She will regard him as a helpful friend if she is not hurt or perplexed by what he says. Deep interpretations are eventually made when the schizophrenic patient's ego has grown stronger and more resilient, as a result of the careful, persistent approach of her Psychoanalyst. The schizophrenic patient's ego is, to start with, frail and with weak boundaries. The early work described above all helps to strengthen it as the patient simultaneously begins to feel more capable and more like herself as she feels she should be, illness aside. When she regards herself as feeling more naturally like a healthy person, she hears her Psychoanalyst make interpretations as well as kind remarks, and she can think for herself in adopting his suggestions for her understanding or discussing these with him. She wants to regain her health, so she makes all the effort she can to respond to whatever he says to her, and if she has difficulty in understanding her Psychoanalyst she knows she can ask directly for further elaboration or explanation. The psychoanalytic psychotherapeutic approach is very versatile, both in making direct, penetrating intercessions into the patient's unconscious mind, and in having full scope also in protecting and supporting the patient as she becomes increasingly well able to learn and implement improvements to her mental health.

An individual's representational world is Joseph Sandler's and Bernard Rosenblatt's psychoanalytic concept of how originally a child or, as later additionally may be considered, an adult, represents in their preconscious mind salient aspects of the environments they have experienced in the past. Their representational world begins to form when the young child notices and experiences features of the world around them and continues to develop accordingly. The representational world gradually changes as the person learns more about the external world, and acts as a guide to them in present and future surroundings to protect and enlighten them about the world around themselves.

It is helpful to the psychoanalytic psychotherapist of schizophrenic and other patients to understand their patient's perspective on the world around them as they proceed in treatment. The patient's attitudes may be explicable in terms of their experiences in the past, and their assumptions and beliefs may also have arisen because of these. If the collective details of the patient's experienced world are assembled together, the Psychoanalyst can place his patient in her context and understand how her feelings may have originated. This becomes very useful to him in working out his approach to resolving her problems, where he can relate his observations and interpretations of her to their source. Feelings can take a long time to resolve; correct attribution allows him to identify them sufficiently clearly to examine them in detail with the patient, and make a start.

The schizophrenic and specifically schizoaffective patient's representational world forms the basis for the PPCC model's initial structuring of her mind at the start of her psychoanalytic psychotherapy (see Chapter 7). The accumulated elements of the patient's world which have contributed to her unpleasant experience of her life thus far can be assembled into the PPCC construct and viewed by the Psychoanalyst as containing this material, or origins of it. He will work with these as he tries to grasp this experience, provide its internal connections in the patient's mind, and help her to acknowledge, address, and adjust to it. He is likely to provide alternative perspectives on to it from her own troubled perceptions, and will try to present a balance of it to her which decreases her painful awareness of it, and consequently a less painful regard towards her present circumstances in the world around her. Despite having grown up within the circumstances of her environments, which produced her preconscious representation of it, she may still be quite unaware of some features which have passed unremarked all her life.

Her Psychoanalyst is in a good position to observe these quietly existing elements and to point out to her their relevance to a positive future which she quite possibly had never contemplated. Her schizophrenic illness will have blinded her to opportunity and blocked out all potential for anything other than its own devastating mental states. Her Psychoanalyst will, when she has partially recovered, make positive comments on her own lateral thinking whenever this occurs, and realistic suggestions in line with nascent hopefulness that she may express. Her representational world is where her mind starts in therapy, containing her past experiences and the details of her past life; her psychoanalytic psychotherapy works with her feelings, her experiences, her dreams and representations, through her observational comments and any meaning that can be gleaned from intermittent psychotic episodes, and brings her to mental health from long before, where she started. Joseph Sandler's and Bernard Rosenblatt's psychoanalytic concept proves extremely useful in psychoanalysing schizophrenic and schizoaffective patients, like others, with psychoanalytic psychotherapy, as much as the practice of classical Psychoanalysis could have done.

Another useful psychoanalytic feature of psychoanalytic psychotherapy is the discipline that classical Psychoanalysis depends upon, of regular sessions. The psychoanalytic 50-minute hour is the optimal length of time for a patient to concentrate on her Psychoanalyst's returns on what she says to him. His interpretations require her to think hard and concentrate on what they mean for her; she can keep up her full effort for this length of time, and wonder, perhaps for her next session, in the remaining 10 minutes what he might have said to her if he had still been present. The time is packed with help, and never quite enough; the patient digests the conversation she has had with him, and thinks about how it connects with the rest of her mind until her ensuing session.

Making the effort to travel to go to see him instils in her the necessity of having to attend her Psychoanalysis sessions. Her sessions come round at a rapid rate, and her physical effort leads to her mental effort in her sessions, to make them worthwhile. Fifty minutes is long enough for a full and meaningful discussion to develop. Sometimes the patient may have difficulty about timing, perhaps thinking if the Psychoanalyst is two minutes late he is ignoring her, or habitually being late in attending her sessions because unconsciously she is avoiding a subject or else her Psychoanalyst himself. The strict timing of the sessions to exactly 50 minutes focuses her mind on what she has to say, with the ends of the sessions actually cutting her off if she has not said the essential meaning she has been trying to communicate to him by then. The absence of niceties at the ends of sessions to some extent protects the Psychoanalyst from social engagement with the patient; his professional role is to discuss with her the issues she raises in connection with her problems as she sees them that have been interfering with her mind. He replies with his psychoanalytic understanding, and in this he very closely tends her mind; but he doesn't have a social relationship with her.

The Psychoanalyst of schizophrenic patients mainly works in his own consulting room, like other Psychoanalysts, but is usually prepared to visit his patient when psychotic in a room on the ward where she is being accommodated due to her being unable to travel to her sessions in his own premises. The sessions will be as strict as in his own office, but she may see a side of him which is different from her regular impressions resulting from her usual routine with him. He will also observe fresh impressions of her which have come to light from her psychosis; she may reveal unfamiliar hostilities, or manifest preoccupations that he did not know about. He might take up Richard Lucas' technique of communicating with her "on the psychotic wavelength" if he thought he could learn about her in this way, or help to reassure her at a particularly difficult time for her. The discipline of her sessions enables the Psychoanalyst to do this and also keeps him apart from her, particularly from her psychosis, which protects him and enables him to treat her psychologically, free from confusion or becoming overly strained.

Non-psychoanalytic features

A non-psychoanalytic feature of psychoanalytic psychotherapy is a requirement for the selection of capable schizophrenic patients able to cope with the great stresses for them of this treatment. Schizophrenic patients are very frail. They are unpredictable, and not able to handle their own minds reliably beyond a basic level. This basic level requires very direct and simple instruction that, utilising their loyalty to the staff and the hospital which may be great, they can follow when their mind is only functioning in an elementary way. Schizophrenic patients do not have common sense. They may see the world very differently even in their lucid state from the norm. Giving a schizophrenic patient the opportunity to undergo psychoanalytic psychotherapy is life-saving for them, and they will nearly always try very hard to do well in it. As a treatment in its early days of development for schizophrenic patients, all the knowledge that is gained about its practice is valuable.

Because schizophrenic patients as a group differ so widely regarding their symptoms and accessibility care needs to be taken not to expect more of them than they can fulfil. They may be too confused; or they may be too despairing; or when very ill they may only be functioning with a basic level of the simplest logic. They are not good at problem-solving, or dealing with truly difficult situations or circumstances. Thinking on their feet, they may fail beyond their capacity to do otherwise, or they may try to act as their confused logic shows them, when their common sense fails. Management of schizophrenic patients in therapy depends on crystal-clear arrangements so that the holes in their minds do not prevail except in the consulting-room. Thinking for themselves will develop within a good transference, which needs to be sustained through the Psychoanalyst's endeavours. Early stages in treatment are the most precarious regarding this, and a patient-centred approach is the best way to maintain contact with the patient when she is beginning to respond to the treatment. If she feels misunderstood or at fault in her new, alarming situation, being psychoanalysed, direct connection with her is the best way to help her. Patients selected for psychoanalytic psychotherapy will all have weaknesses where they fall down. Their dependability and the dependability of the staff, amounting to loyalty to each other, is the best foundation for the treatment.

In some parts of the world physical restraint is used to control patients whose behaviour cannot otherwise be managed. This is disappointing for everyone. Classical Psychoanalysis has never countenanced physical restraint of its patients, and psychoanalytic psychotherapy would never normally engage with it either. On a hospital ward patients sometimes become very distressed; patients can communicate distress to each other, and if this happens staff may find managing the ward challenging until peace is restored. Talking to a patient appeals to their humanity and common sense, and nurse therapists who mainly supervise ward management are brave and committed individuals who bring out the best in their patients but also have to tackle disturbances in this way. In the UK physical restraint is rarely used, especially on psychotherapy wards, because here the better part of the patients' selves is appealed to, and generally they respond well. Injections of a sedative such as chlorpromazine, or diazepam in less aroused cases, is the usual method of physical restraint. The first approach is to give oral medication, which is less disturbing both for the patient and the atmosphere on the ward if the medicine can be taken this way. Psychodynamic understanding of psychosis, and regular ward groups on a daily basis, maintains a psychotherapy ward in its ideal state. This can be attained with sufficient staff who are well looked after themselves and enjoy their work, so that every communication is attuned to the patients' wellbeing. On such a ward physical restraint is rarely required. In this environment, schizophrenic patients may be supervised in a state of wellbeing while their mental state is steadily improving with their psychoanalytic psychotherapy. Disturbance on the ward interferes with this progress, and certainly physical restraint becomes a setback for them if it ever has to be resorted to.

Family therapy is an aspect of the overall treatment of schizophrenic patients advocated by Dr Michael Robbins in his hierarchy of eight systems (see Chapter 7) which is based around psychoanalytic psychotherapy. Family therapy was never a part of Freud's classical psychoanalytic practice. When a schizophrenic patient undergoes psychoanalytic psychotherapy that enables her to emerge as herself out of her illness condition, her family may be none the wiser about this. They may not understand at all what her treatment has consisted of, nor how she will have changed, possibly out of all recognition of herself as a very afflicted schizophrenic individual. In order that she may continue to progress, her family will need to recognise her newly developed capacities, such as her ability to articulate, her independent thinking, her autonomy, and how they should relate to her in view of these. It may be hard for them to accept these changes in her, and to treat her with renewed kindness and respect. Strong feelings may be aroused in family therapy. These need to be contained within the family therapy group by the psychoanalytic psychotherapy clinician who is treating the patient, and usually another member of staff who attends it, supporting him in their task together. Giving the patient space to speak to her family in the family therapy group with her new-found individuation, autonomy, and independence is very therapeutic for her; it may be one of the first places where she becomes able to exercise herself as she wishes to be, with other people. The two clinicians support her in her new position and try to prevent hard feelings becoming established in the family. If the patient finds herself unable to make her new circumstance clear to her relatives, she may decide to leave the family environment, but on as good terms as possible.

Classical Psychoanalysis as practised by Freud did not suggest methods of working with psychotic symptoms. Even today, though some following Richard Lucas' idea of communicating with patients when psychotic may do so, patients in a psychotic state are generally cared for in hospital until the psychosis subsides, when they resume sessions with their Psychoanalyst in his consulting room. Psychoanalysts since the earliest days have tried to understand schizophrenia, and developed theories to explain it. Classical Psychoanalysis cannot explain specific psychotic symptoms, nor provide exclusively within its own methodology a means of treating it; the schizophrenic patient cannot handle simple interpretations on their own, even if the Psychoanalyst has his own theories about what is going on in his patient's mind, based on previous Psychoanalysts' work. The patient requires support during the session, which psychoanalytic psychotherapy supplies; the Psychoanalyst confirms the patient in her observations where he can, empathises with her, reassures her where this is warranted, and gives her all the time she needs to work out and endure her feelings while she responds to his latest comment on what she herself has said. Progress may be slow, but all the time that is spent in this way reinforces the patient's experience of herself in an unthreatening environment where her true, authentic attitudes and her own meanings have a chance to be discovered by her. It seems to be true in schizophrenic illness that the patient rarely volunteers what she really feels in a meaningful way;

she does not have good enough relationships with anyone where she can discuss this with them. Her unpleasant experiences have crushed it out of her, and usually she has become turned inwards, away from the world, introverted, and very sad. Psychoanalytic psychotherapy offers her a way to reverse this, with the support she needs, based as it is on Freud's classical psychoanalytic technique. Sometimes the Psychoanalyst needs to stimulate her, mildly provocatively, if she remains withdrawn in her sessions, to elicit manifestly her responses to him; and this encouragement from time to time will assist her in making steady progress.

References

Freud, S (1911). Psycho-analytic notes on an autobiographical account of a case of paranoia (Dementia Paranoides). In *The Standard Edition of the Complete Psychological Works of Sigmund Freud*, Ed. Strachey, J. Vol.XII, pp.3–82. London: Vintage (2001).

Robbins, M (1993). *Experiences of Schizophrenia: An Integration of the Personal, Scientific and Therapeutic.* New York: Guilford Press.

Shedler, J (2010). The efficiency of psychodynamic psychotherapy. *American Psychologist*, 65(2):98–109.

Steggles, G (2019). *The Psychiatry of Resolving Schizophrenia Psychoanalytically: How Visualising the Therapeutic Process Can Assist Success.* UK: Free Association Books.

Zetzel, E (1970). The capacity for emotional growth. *The International Psycho-Analytical Library No. 86.* Toronto: Hogarth Press.

Chapter 6

Psychotherapeutic approaches to schizophrenia

Psychotherapy is a general term for a clinician's approach to a distressed individual when the therapy proceeds through conversation. Common to all psychotherapies is the supportive approach; the therapist tries to strengthen the patient in her weakness, with his selection from a variety of emphases and techniques that he thinks are best suited to his patient's needs. Psychotherapy can be very effective. Some forms of psychotherapy are best suited to particular types of problem, such as psychodynamic psychotherapy for psychotic conditions and cognitive behaviour therapy (CBT) for practical or psychological bad habits that a patient may have fallen into; psychoanalytic psychotherapy is one of the best treatments for schizophrenia but is also widely used when radical change in a patient is needed to structure their future life. Some authorities such as Andrew Lewis (Lewis, 2008) advocate an integrated psychotherapeutic model for the treatment of psychosis; but this volume herein emphasises the clarity which may be achieved by establishing precise clinical technique in working with the patient, in using accurately guiding theoretical models, and in working only, in these treatments, with those patients who have their own incentive to overcome the difficulties in mentalising to which their circumstances and previous environments have restricted them.

Patients who have a psychogenic schizophrenia secondary to trauma or to adverse circumstances and involving psychotic defence mechanisms, and who have already achieved significantly, earlier in life, may recover substantive mentalising capacities. Intense, precise therapeutic work is able to identify defence mechanisms, and hence potentially to restore mentalisation. All psychotherapy needs to be kind to the patient; however, it is not kind nor helpful to expose a patient to therapeutic situations which they can neither understand, on

DOI: 10.4324/9781003433507-9

top of their existing difficulties due to illness, nor are able to act upon in their own interests. In cases where the therapist cannot achieve his aims with his patient, impasse is reached because he cannot help them further, and the therapy is terminated. Therefore the challenges of psychoanalytic psychotherapy are very carefully and with caution offered to a prospective, hopeful patient, perhaps commencing only with a trial period of six months before commitment to an entire treatment.

Psychotherapy can adopt individual, group, and community approaches. Aspects of individual work with patients will mainly be discussed here; groups offer more general support and also a chance for social interaction among patients. It seems that compromised schizophrenic patients themselves, and their families particularly, value the Open Dialogue and Need-Adapted community approach originating in Finland, where what they say is taken at face value, and they learn from discussions with each other and the leaders of the community groups. Articulating self-truths meaningfully is key, after all, to most talking therapies. Accepting also its mechanism as brain dysfunction, psychosis is seen generally as the mind's understandable, reactive way of dealing with the unbearable, which considered psychodynamic understanding addresses more specifically and realistically. And avoiding stress in the psychotherapeutic communities is found by many to be important to their progress. Psychodynamic psychotherapy in psychotherapeutic communities such as the Turku Schizophrenia Project in Finland achieves good results for severely ill patients; following time spent on the psychotherapeutic ward, some patients are allocated a therapist and pursue individual psychodynamically oriented psychotherapy with them (Alanen, 1997). Open Dialogue and Need-Adapted treatments in Finland involve families in therapy to ease the development of the patient's future relationships using their new, therapy-derived skills.

In the MacLean Hospital, Massachusetts, where Dr Michael Robbins worked, two different forms of individual psychotherapy were compared by other clinicians. Explorative, insight-oriented (EIO) psychotherapy and Reality-Adaptive, Supportive (RAS) psychotherapy were compared in a study which showed similar results for each method, though these have not, since, become widely used. Dr Robbins' own work remains the clearest exposition of a successful method of addressing the problems faced in treating schizophrenic patients, and his own approach to psychoanalytic psychotherapy with them illustrates a rate of success that has not been bettered. Those patients given the opportunity of psychoanalytic psychotherapy face a lot of stress in different ways, but potentially also may reap its benefits.

Psychodynamic psychotherapy

Psychodynamics is the study of mental and emotional forces affecting the mind, arising from past experiences and leading to effects on the patient. When these mental and emotional forces arise from elements the mind considers unacceptable to the individual, they may initiate a psychotic process in the individual. This psychotic process involves expelling the element into the outside world, often into other people, which may have pathological consequences; the mind may alternatively repress the unwanted element down into its own unconscious, where it can initiate a neurotic illness. Psychodynamic understanding may elucidate the form and nature of these psychotic and neurotic processes affecting the patient so that she may be treated psychoanalytically.

It is widely held that the personality is sometimes particularly vulnerable to stresses from outside which necessitate it defending itself from them. Zubin and Spring introduced the stress-vulnerability nomenclature in 1977 when they produced their stress-vulnerability model (Zubin et al., 1977). Here the emphasis was on the episodic course of schizophrenia, contrasting this with a continuous disease process. They believed that each episode was precipitated by endogenous and exogenous challenging events which exceeded the patient's vulnerability threshold. Zubin and Spring argued that vulnerability is either a genetically or, by contrast, an environmentally acquired level of risk for developing the illness; this could be counteracted by coping abilities and by a capacity to learn from the experiences of previous episodes. This theory has been extended by Read and colleagues' traumagenic neurodevelopmental model (Read et al., 2001) which substitutes trauma for the idea of stress (Lewis, 2008).

These theories' shared concept is that when trauma or stresses threaten the integrity of a person's mind it needs to take fundamental action to prevent itself fragmenting and disintegrating. Sometimes the stress or trauma is so severe that the mind resorts to a psychotic defence, which may in itself precipitate its own fragmentation and disintegration if the person is sufficiently vulnerable to this. There are many defence mechanisms; over 100 have been listed by Jerome Blackman (Blackman, 2004). Only some of these are manifest in psychosis rather than in neurosis, however, and a familiar handful recur repeatedly and commonly in psychotic illness. Projective identification has been recognised often as being a substantial part of schizophrenic pathology, including by Freud, Klein, and Bion. Splitting, where another person's good and bad attributes or any other contrasted aspects are completely separated in a person's mind, is thought to occur first in tiny babies adjusting to the presence of their mother, and to continue throughout life but particularly in schizophrenic psychosis. Denial occurs in all of us as we try to protect ourselves from unpleasantness, fearful consequences, or accusations; psychotic illness is not necessary for its employment.

Recognising defence mechanisms in a psychotic patient's presentation can provide a key to understanding what her mind has been trying to protect, and hence enlighten the core of her psychotic illness. Even if only one episode of illness can be understood at a time, cumulatively the patient may begin to feel she herself is in safe hands, and her illness could be understood so that she can live her life more peacefully.

Brian Martindale's excellent paper (Martindale, 2007) "Psychodynamic contributions to early intervention in psychosis" elucidates all these points clearly, and makes a plea for psychodynamics to be utilised by early intervention teams who are, increasingly, young people's first line of contact at the onset of illness. "Understanding" makes a great difference to the mentally ill, and sometimes politics can interfere with good patient care. He writes, in 2007, that psychodynamics is rarely integrated into the Psychiatry of psychosis when it could bestow so much relief to those whom interventions serve. Sharing knowledge and taking proper responsibility can achieve good results, especially when the knowledge is so lucid and efficacious. Martindale's paper is replete with examples of the lucidity of psychodynamics and therefore of its potential usefulness to patient care.

The schizoaffective patient around whose clinical case the PPCC model was built (see Chapter 7) was a young woman who in the early stages of her illness had specific psychotic symptoms. These demonstrated psychotic defence mechanisms and can be seen (below) to be psychogenic in origin, thus offering support for the theories of reactive schizophrenia or schizoaffective disorder described above. The patient had been severely sexually traumatised by her father as a child, followed by major family upheaval and unpleasantness. Psychoanalytic psychotherapy utilising a minimum of necessary medication under Psychiatric care completely resolved her illness.

Two psychotic symptoms will be described, followed by identification of the defence mechanisms operating and the psychodynamic processes involved.

Vignette 1

The patient had been upset by a remark of her father's that belittled the genuine act of kindness she was in the process of preparing, in the form of a golden wedding anniversary cake for her grandparents. He had, unwittingly or carelessly, belittled her previously on a number of occasions, sometimes after special effort but on one occasion simply on the basis of her biological development, seen by him as tardy.

That night, in the darkness of the early hours, she hallucinated a black psychopath crouching outside her bedroom window, which was terrifyingly trying to control her as she lay in her bed by speaking into a microphone; though she heard no words.

The patient had split her father's kindness from his clumsy, insensitive comments and his molestation of her. She projectively identified with the black psychopath by sending all her worst feelings about her father into it. Martindale's view is that it is important to pay attention to the content of delusions and hallucinations "for clues as to the very personal nature of 'toxic' stresses" (Martindale, 2007). The wicked figure in the hallucination symbolically represented her father speaking (albeit silently) to her; its intolerable presence replicated the presence of her father, which she found unbearable.

In their 2013 paper "The psychodynamics of psychosis" Brian Martindale and Alison Summers suggest that we can consider psychosis as "a response to unbearable aspects of reality" (Martindale et al., 2013). The patient was under a lot of stress relating to the family's problems, as well as her stressed relationship with her father and demanding studies. When her feelings were hurt again, relating to her grandparents' cake, the reality known to her became unbearable. The common factor of her father as agent in the remarks and her sexual trauma was the connection between the trigger for the psychosis involving the cake and the form and content of the hallucination. The psychogenesis of the hallucination is clear to see.

Martindale also writes, in "Psychodynamic contributions to early intervention in psychosis":

> When psychogenic factors are at work in psychosis, psychodynamics conceives of the unconscious mind as trying to expel from itself aspects of internal or external reality that are too unbearable, too unacceptable, or too overwhelming, so that the person carries on as if aspects of reality did not exist.
>
> (Martindale, 2007, p.36)
> (Reproduced with permission of Cambridge
> University Press through PLSclear)

Accordingly, the psychodynamics of the hallucination emphasise the expulsion of the patient's memory of her unbearable, unacceptable, overwhelming sexual assault into a figment of her imagination, her mind's hallucination of a dark figure. She carried on with her life trying to block out her father's existence for years before her very strained attitude towards, and feeling for, her father was resolved through psychoanalytic psychotherapy.

Symptomatically, the patient's sleep paralysis experience involved a visual hallucination; a "potential" auditory hallucination ("speaking" into a microphone in order to control the patient, but without any words); and a delusion of control of the patient by the visually hallucinated figure, which mirrored the control of the patient by her father during the sexual trauma. The experience can largely be explained psychogenically, and psychodynamics provides clear evidence of the strength and nature of the feeling with which the patient regarded her father.

Vignette 2

The patient "saw" a Chinese mandarin on her psychiatric ward. But she reasoned that no Chinese mandarin would ever be housed on a psychiatric ward, so the figure must be a dressed-up actor.

In fact, a young male nurse had acquired an adventurous coiffure with his head shaven except for a high ponytail, conveying an Eastern impression like that in one of the patient's childhood picture books.

Here the patient is demonstrating concretisation; she could not contemplate abstractly any everyday person looking like that on the ward; she concluded with a defensive, physical explanation, that she was looking at a Chinese mandarin. Then she intellectualised; there could not be a real Chinese mandarin on the psychiatric ward. She rationalised freshly that the individual must be an actor. And finally, she generalised that "there must be actors on the ward".

Martindale and Summers write, in "The psychodynamics of psychosis":

> In psychodynamic approaches to all mental phenomena there is emphasis not only on impressions of external reality but also on changes in processing of psychic or internal emotional reality. These changes help the mind create a more acceptable view of itself and its intersubjective reality, and are mostly in broad accordance with the views of others (these are the defence mechanisms of the non-psychotic part of the personality). Sometimes, however, the mind creates "a new reality" that is more acceptable to it but which is outside the sphere of "common sense" (this is the functioning of a psychotic part of the personality).
>
> (Martindale et al., 2013, p.124)
> (Reproduced with permission of Cambridge University Press through PLSclear)

In this instance, there were several changes in the processing of the patient's psychic reality. Here, the impression of external reality considered psychodynamically was of looking at a Chinese mandarin. This made the patient feel awkward and vulnerable, bending to the mandarin's superiority. A more acceptable and friendly view for herself and her situation, a "new reality", was to be surrounded by actors on the ward. Initially, therefore, she had a delusional perception that she was looking at a Chinese mandarin; and second, her defence mechanisms led to a further delusion, that she was surrounded by actors, which was much more comfortable than being exposed to the presence of a Chinese mandarin.

Freud in 1924 wrote that, in the case of schizophrenia:

the delusion is found applied like a patch over the place where originally a rent had appeared in the ego's relation to the external world. If this pre-condition of a conflict with the external world is not much more noticeable to us than it now is, that is because, in the clinical picture of the psychosis, the manifestations of the pathogenic process are often overlaid by manifestations of an attempt at a cure or a reconstruction.

(Freud, 1924, p.151)

In our example, the attempt at a cure was to populate the ward with actors, to cope with the rent in the patient's ego's relation to the external world, i.e. the shock and intimidation accompanying the presence of the mistakenly but credulously perceived Chinese mandarin.

In summary, the psychodynamic view is that the content of psychotic symptoms is meaningful (Martindale et al., 2013). In our examples, the black psychopath meaningfully reflected the patient's horrified feelings in relation to her father. And the patient on the ward experienced much more ongoing comfort in her life when believing she was surrounded by actors rather than in the presence of a Chinese mandarin.

Martindale and Summers also write, in "The psychodynamics of psychosis":

In the psychodynamic approach to psychosis, attention is paid to clarifying experiences of reality that the person has found unmanageable and which have, through psychosis, been dispensed with or altered, rather than contained, "digested" and integrated as in non-psychotic states. Once the anxieties, disintegration and emotional pain underlying the psychosis are understood, the psychosis may be seen to have a self-preservation and even a developmental function.

(Martindale et al., 2013, pp.124–5)
(Reproduced with permission of Cambridge
University Press through PLSclear)

Freud's "patch" over a mental "rent" can certainly be seen to have its self-preserving role in the mind of this patient trying to survive after her major trauma. She was reminded by the black psychopath to stay away from people frighteningly trying to control her. And she regained a sense of comfort after a startling observation by reflecting on more benign even if unrealistic companions on her psychiatric ward.

Cognitive Behaviour Therapy

CBT has been recently adapted to the treatment of psychosis; its proponents advocate a symptom-based approach (Hagen et al., 2011). This utilises cognitive models of psychosis, based on the concept of discrete symptoms better reflecting the evidence of a continuity between mental illness and mental health and between the "psychotic" and the "normal" than do discrete diagnostic classificatory systems for psychosis. It does remain true, however, that accurate diagnosis is important for prognosis, and also for the usefulness of specific treatments for a particular individual. CBT may be selected as a mode of treatment, but for the patient's future safety a provisional diagnosis should be made. This is especially important for a psychotic patient, since the choice of medication can make a great difference to how she is empowered to manage herself when away from Psychiatric care. Her illness is too serious to allow its management to be vague.

Hagen and colleagues write about three paradigms that have been distinguished historically in our understanding of psychosis: the illness paradigm introduced by Kraepelin (Kraepelin, 1893), where diagnosable mental illnesses were considered to be brain disorders; the stress vulnerability model (Zubin et al., 1977), where biologically and psychologically predisposed individuals may become psychotic if they are exposed to stressful life experiences; and the symptom-focused paradigm, where each symptom is emphasised rather than using broad diagnostic categories (Hagen et al., 2011).

The CBT of psychosis can be divided into five phases related to therapeutic processes taking place between the patient and the therapist. Initially, the focus is on engaging the patient in a therapeutic alliance. Then the aim is to educate and normalise the patient's psychotic symptoms; the therapist tries to demonstrate other examples of ordinary psychological phenomena similar to the patient's symptoms, trying to help her feel listened to and understood. After this stage, the therapist and patient develop and share a case formulation together. Based on this a treatment plan is made, that works with the patient's beliefs and thoughts related to her understanding of her symptoms and trying to build new alternative explanations and coping strategies. The aim is not to make the psychotic symptoms go away but to restructure previous views of voices and delusions and to generate new, less distressing ones. The intention is to lessen the patient's emotional distress. The conclusion of the treatment is to achieve relapse prevention and recovery.

CBT has not widely been taken up as a method of treating psychosis. Developing a cognitive mini-formulation of delusional thoughts may make sense to the patient, but as a cognitive memory itself is likely to fade with time. CBT in its wider practice has been found to be effective initially but gradually to become less effective in its role of preventing symptoms. Psychosis is deep-rooted in the psyche; it emerges from the unconscious, and is thought to originate in the oldest parts of the brain where emotions are usually regulated, the limbic system. Cognition arises from the phylogenetically newer cortex of the brain, and is conscious. The newer cortex does not exert much control over the older parts of the brain. Therefore, treatment affecting consciousness and cognition, CBT, may make cognitive sense to the patient, but does not affect or stop the more basic processes of psychosis. Treatments that access the unconscious, such as psychoanalytic psychotherapy, have a chance of calming the unconscious mind, reaching the older parts of the brain, especially over time in a treatment lasting a number of years. Courses of CBT are traditionally short, and may help in the short term, but its conscious memories are not long-lasting and so cannot resolve the origin of a patient's psychosis.

Need-Adapted treatment

This form of psychotherapy emphasises intensity, versatility, and teamwork, with "a basic psychotherapeutic attitude". It was developed in the 1980s and is based in Turku, in south-west Finland (Alanen, 1997). It features psychotherapeutic communities, and is developed from standard hospital wards, family therapeutic sessions, and individual therapeutic relationships. There is an emphasis on an empathic attitude, open communication, the development of therapeutic relationships with a patient's personal nurse within the therapeutic communities, family therapeutic activities, and the support of the patient's continuing contacts outside the hospital ward. Individual therapy is psychodynamically oriented, and better results have been unsurprisingly found with better-trained staff than with inexperienced nurses; with these the number of inpatient days per year were found to decrease. With family therapy, likewise, the psychotic symptoms of many patients disappeared or quickly decreased; hospital admissions became much shorter.

General principles of Need-Adapted treatment (Alanen, 1997, pp.171–3) include provision that:

- Therapeutic activities are planned and carried out flexibly and individually in each case.
- Examination and treatment are dominated by a psychotherapeutic attitude.
- Different therapeutic approaches should supplement each other rather than constituting an either/or approach.
- The treatment should attain the quality of a continuous process.
- Follow-up of the individual patients and of the efficacy of the treatment methods is important for evaluation and future development of services.

All five principles of Need-Adapted treatment are necessary for its effective implementation.

(Reproduced with permission of Informa UK Limited through PLSclear)

Need-Adapted treatment is patient-centred. Shared mental representation guiding the therapeutic process is a prerequisite for achieving integrated treatment of schizophrenia. Patients' needs change: Yrjo Alanen and colleagues' concept of "need-specific treatment" was adjusted and changed to "Need-Adapted treatment". Shared understanding between the patient, her family and the clinical staff was the objective, but not to reach the patient's unconscious mind in order to get to the root cause of the psychosis; there was no emphasis on the difference between constitutional schizophrenia which had steadily developed since birth and reactive schizophrenia that appeared to be a clinical response to very unpleasant environmental experiences lived through during development.

The recovery from a regressive psychotic state brought about in Turku by early and intensive family-centred treatment was found to occupy a key role in the further treatment of schizophrenic patients in community Psychiatry. Long-term individual psychotherapy was also found to benefit patients considerably. Another clear finding was that being in a marital relationship at the onset of illness led to a better prognosis upon resolution of the psychotic symptoms. It was also found, in common with many other psychological treatments, that women had a better prognosis than men.

Comparisons of the psychotherapies for schizophrenia

Psychodynamic psychotherapy utilises Freud's concept of the unconscious mind for understanding psychotic defences. Clinicians who have studied this approach become very skilled in understanding the utterances of patients when they are psychotic, after they have worked at analysing them and tried to make sense of them. This skill is particularly useful in early intervention interviews when a Psychiatrist tends a young person during his or her first psychotic episode; if sense can be made when the young person first tries to communicate what is upsetting him or her, the clinician is in an advantageous position to make the best arrangements for the patient. The duration of untreated psychosis is known to be highly influential in the recovery time needed for the young person; if what they have been trying to express is received appropriately and he or she is responded to accordingly, then the worst aspects from the patient's point of view will have been transferred to safe hands. For other patients, the symbolism of their psychotic defences may be picked up by the skilled psychodynamic therapist and interpreted in terms of the situation the patient may have left just prior to admission. This symbolism can reveal the nature of the circumstances that have recently upset the patient – who may indeed have a psychotic illness that requires medication – and notwithstanding the patient's possibly general state of confusion, the specific trigger for this episode may be neutralised for her. In doing so, this may considerably calm her.

Need-Adapted treatment is a very broad approach. It does not study the patient's mind so much as assist her functioning, in the family and socially, as a member of these communities. This is a great contrast to CBT, which addresses not only the patient's mind itself but specific symptoms. The basis for the Need-Adapted approach seems to be the context of the family, not considering the individual person isolated in the world at large, trying to function autonomously, but helping her to fit in with other people. The treatment is not aiming for individual change, but rather integration with others in a continuous process as the person she is, hoping the psychosis will subside with the therapy rather than tackling its causes.

These two psychotherapies, CBT and Need-Adapted treatment, differ substantially from psychoanalytic psychotherapy. Here the therapy addresses specifically the patient's manifest symptoms and complaints, and interprets these increasingly deeply, aiming to reach her unconscious core where her mind suffers emotional disturbance relating to early experiences and memories: drawing these to her attention allows her to understand herself in them, at the times they happened, and her subsequent responses. Once she can recognise her past's reality, with her experiences' now-understandable origins, her emotions are likely to stabilise in her Psychoanalyst's care. Then her social relationships may strengthen her in her new perspectives and experience of herself, whether or not she retains contact with her family of birth. This treatment gives the patient full scope to emerge out of her previous circumstances and develop for herself individuation of the kind, as far as it is possible to see, that she might well have developed had she never been ill. This is a remarkable achievement for the Psychoanalyst, for the patient, and for the potential of the treatment; successes of this kind may then be applied to further patients with schizophrenia or schizoaffective disorder.

Explorative, Insight-Orientated (EIO), and Reality-Adaptive, Supportive (RAS) psychotherapies are two forms of psychotherapy which were practised with schizophrenic patients in MacLean Hospital in Massachusetts, the same centre where Dr Michael Robbins practised psychoanalytic psychotherapy. They were assessed in a study aimed at comparing the two individual therapy approaches. Appropriate doses of medication were also given. Explorative, Insight-Orientated psychotherapy, as its name suggests, encouraged an inward-looking perspective in its patients, helping them to learn about themselves and their own experiences. Reality-Adaptive, Supportive psychotherapy attempted to enable patients to relate better to external conditions, in the outside world around them. When results from the two methods of psychotherapy were compared, no great difference was found between them. At the two-year follow-up the EIO patients were found to have improved more regarding their thought disorder, whereas the RAS patients' social functioning and especially performance at work was clearly better than for the EIO patients. Psychodynamic exploration during EIO therapy helped alleviate some symptoms, although anxiety and depression surfaced upon the patients' emerging from their apathy and isolation; this differed from patients in RAS therapy, where active support given by therapists correlated with a decrease of anxiety and depression. Neither EIO nor RAS forms of psychotherapy were taken up in other centres, possibly because inward-looking and externally focused scrutiny are both needed for a patient to become mentally adjusted and well in the environments they move in. Depending upon either one of these at the expense of the other does not leave the patient equipped to live their life, functioning fully.

Motivational interviewing is a brief form of psychotherapy where the clinician encourages the patient to discuss her plans with her own drive and enthusiasm. The only initiative apparent during the interview is that of the patient. The interviewer reinforces what the patient says, and asks questions about the attitudes and feelings expressed by the patient. He agrees with what the patient says, and gives encouragement to her ideas and hopes, helping the patient to clarify and determine her future actions. The interviewer expresses empathy with the patient and draws to her attention the discrepancy between her behaviours and her values; awareness of this can increase her motivation to change. Rather as with CBT, the schizophrenic patient will be helped to change what she can about her present life through cognitive effort. The interviewer asks open-ended questions and uses the patient's reflections on these to help her draw a picture of the future she sees for herself. More than the Psychoanalyst's evenly suspended positive regard, the motivational interviewer reflectively listens, but also encourages the patient in her choices, which a Psychoanalyst would never do. The interviewer affirms the patient's decisions, and encourages her and supports her during the change process. Towards the end of the process the interviewer summarises his discussion with the patient, and having resolved residual ambivalence, tries to strengthen the patient's commitment to plans they have discussed and to actions she intends to take. The schizophrenic patient's ability to respond to motivational interviewing may be limited, but within her capacity she may be willing to try harder to function effectively in her life rather than give in despondently to her situation; her self-care and social arrangements may improve following motivational interviewing with a compassionate care worker.

References

Alanen, Y (1997). *Schizophrenia: Its Origins and Need-Adapted Treatment.* pp.171–3. London: Karnac. Reproduced with permission of Informa UK Limited through PLSclear.

Blackman, J (2004). *101 Defences: How the Mind Shields Itself.* Hove: Brunner-Routledge.

Freud, S (1924). Neurosis and psychosis. In: *The Standard Edition of the Complete Psychological Works of Sigmund Freud*, Ed. Strachey, J. Vol. XIX, p.151. London: Vintage (2001).

Hagen, R; Turkington. D; Berge, T; Grawe, R (2011). *CBT for Psychosis: A Symptom-Based Approach.* Hove: Routledge.

Kraepelin, E (1893). *Dementia Praecox and Paraphrenia.* Pub. Edinburgh: Livingstone (1919).

Lewis, Andrew (2008). Neuropsychological deficit and psychodynamic defence models of schizophrenia: Towards an integrated psychotherapeutic model. In: *Psychotherapies for the Psychoses: Theoretical, Cultural and Clinical Integration.* Eds. Gleeson, J; Killackey, E; Krstev, H. pp.52–69. Hove: Routledge.

Martindale, B (2007). Psychodynamic contributions to early intervention in psychosis. *Advances in Psychiatric Treatment*, **13**: 13–42. Reproduced with permission of Cambridge University Press through PLSclear.

Martindale, B; Summers, A (2013). The psychodynamics of psychosis. *Advances in Psychiatric Treatment*, 19: 124–31. Reproduced with permission of Cambridge University Press through PLSclear.

Read, J; Perry, B; Moskowitz, A; Connolly, J (2001). The contribution of early traumatic events to schizophrenia in some patients. A traumagenic neurodevelopmental model. *Psychiatry: Interpersonal and Biological Processes*, 64: 319–345.

Zubin, J; Spring, B (1977). Vulnerability: A new view of schizophrenia. *Journal of Abnormal Psychology*, 86: 103–26.

Part III

The process and results of treating schizophrenic and schizoaffective patients with psychoanalytic psychotherapy

Chapter 7

Effective hospital-based treatment of schizophrenic patients

Schizophrenia and schizoaffective disorder are extremely serious illnesses which completely disrupt affected patients' lives. They both comprise forms of psychosis which overwhelm the sufferer, in acute attacks of illness which render the patient quite helpless and instigate long periods of suffering deeply unpleasant mental states that are beyond description or parallel. Hospitalisation is required while they are in a helpless state, but is kept to the minimum necessary; staying with relatives or their own or hostel accommodation is the usual solution while they are learning to tolerate their new situation of having to cope effectively with their illness. Current hospital treatment of schizophrenic patients is managed by Consultant Psychiatrists who have trained in Adult and Community Psychiatry; but if on his hospital ward is housed a schizophrenic patient who is receiving psychoanalytic psychotherapy, the ward Psychiatrist will also have a good knowledge of Psychoanalysis so that he can supervise his patient's therapy by her Psychiatry-trained Psychoanalyst. These two clinicians liaise closely in her care and both are alert to changes in her as she progresses through her treatment.

Hospital care

When patients are experiencing acute attacks of psychosis they are quite unable to look after themselves; hospital care is the only safe solution for them. The life-long distress which a diagnosis of schizophrenia without treatment entails is endured by the patient no matter what other factors prevail. For untreated patients elements of confusion and distress remain with them for the rest of their lives, and they tolerate these throughout all their activities and experiences generally,

DOI: 10.4324/9781003433507-11

whatever the pattern of their lives, whoever they spend time with, no matter what their preferences might be. The illness affects most areas of mental functioning; patients differ in their combinations of symptoms. Sometimes the stress of it all proves too much, and some sufferers do not feel they can survive.

For these reasons, everything possible is done for schizophrenic patients who come to Health Services' notice. The usual pattern is for hospitalisation while the patient is comforted and reassured that they will receive the help available, and medication specific to their needs as far as this can effectively be selected is arranged by their ward Psychiatrist, who tailors it accurately with maximum control of the patient's symptoms and minimum causation of side-effects. Taking medication of any kind is not pleasant; psychotic patients' disturbed states of mind can interfere with their co-operation with ward staff because of anxieties or even fears, old prejudices, mistaken assumptions, and quite commonly anger at having control taken away from them relating to their most personal needs and functions. Ward staff work very hard to ensure patients feel secure and comforted wherever this can be achieved. The patient finding themselves in a psychiatric ward, uprooted from their home, in addition to the shock of their own symptoms which they absolutely cannot understand, characteristically takes many days or weeks to stabilise, and this is among other patients in similar or even worse states. The ward Psychiatrist supervises and guides the staff on his ward as they supervise the patients in their care; he carries responsibility for everything that happens there, keeping in close touch with patients' progress and staff wellbeing.

The ward Charge Nurse or Sister, and perhaps a Deputy Sister also, ensure that all the ward staff know and understand their roles relating to patient care. On a psychotherapy ward, every communication should be in harmony with the ward ambience to ensure that patient progress is a continuous process with as few setbacks as possible. Raised voices or forgetfulness or rushing about should not occur; all of these will disturb the patients and distract them from their own tasks regarding their thinking. Psychotherapy patients learn to concentrate on themselves in a good psychotherapy ward. Those receiving individual psychotherapy or Psychoanalysis will be trying to make sense of themselves, with varying degrees of success. The only reason they are there is because in some way they have been unable to do so at a fundamental level which has required intervention, with questions asked about themselves: and these they know they have to answer.

Kind staff make this task more palatable, even fun with a lighter side to the ward; the pain and difficulties become more bearable.

Regular psychodynamic groups, daily if possible and even more than one on some days in the week, provide opportunities for connections between the patients and staff and between the patients themselves. This all helps the cohesion of the ward as a psychotherapy unit. Interpretations during the groups, and those made at other times by individual staff members during daily incidental conversations with the patients, repeatedly remind them about issues they have with their minds. Everything that happens on the ward is arranged to make this introspection a regular practice with each patient. In time, this becomes a habit which the patients practise, continuously sometimes, for years after leaving the ward; this is very often necessary for them to maintain their progress by observing for themselves their faulty mental habits which they try to counteract using the learned good habits. It will generally have taken a lifetime for their mind to develop as it has, with its faults, bad habits, and tendencies, and the patient may spend the rest of their life, educated on the psychotherapy ward, trying to reverse the process. The camaraderie on the ward among both patients and staff colour this with optimism, so the patients tend to set off home with a will. Good practice needs to be shared widely so that far more patients distressed by illness can be shown the way to manage their conditions.

Ward psychodynamic groups, attended by all ward patients, are opportunities for the staff to make general psychodynamic interpretations, which may be psychoanalytic in character, about issues that have come to light during the day. Patients' unconscious minds become engaged in what is said, and each patient reflects for themselves and learns from its relevance for them. Dark areas that each patient brings to the ward have a chance of surfacing in the groups, presented in the patient's best light, open to comments from everyone attending. These sessions, together with individual psychotherapy, medication, occupational therapy, family therapy, and close supervision on the ward by the staff, constitute the ideal milieu for resolving serious and debilitating experiences of mental illness.

Psychodynamic family therapy is undertaken to understand the schizophrenic patient's family systemically, and to help her to become re-established within it once they have adjusted their attitudes and responses to her in her new, psychologically maturing state. They may have to take particular care to treat her kindly and with respect, perhaps after years of not understanding her at all, or certainly as she would like to have been understood. During family therapy, strong feelings may be aroused; resentment and even anger may emerge, which fall on to the Psychoanalyst running the small group, and his trained assistant from the ward staff, to contain. Sometimes the family work well together, allowance is made in different ways, and the Psychoanalyst's insightful points, difficult for them to hear, are received with acceptance. If the ensuing tensions are too great, the patient may decide to leave the family, but on the best terms possible.

Patient safety

Patient safety is widely held to be the single most important aspect of clinical care. Schizophrenic patients have a particularly complex disorder, and their predictability becomes less certain than that of other patients in their day-to-day management because of this. Their true motivations and intentions may remain hidden due to powerful defences, so ward staff must remain vigilant and know their whereabouts at all times, especially if they travel from hospital to see their Psychoanalyst and back; timing and communicating their departure at either end allows an alert to be signalled should any mishap occur. Good relationships with the ward staff help to promote loyalty in the patient to them, to the ward and to the hospital. The patient's sense of loyalty, however ill they are, is one of the greatest assets the staff can promote in the cause of keeping the patient safe, in every sense.

When the patient is too ill to visit her Psychoanalyst, he will usually visit her on the ward. If he is concerned about her after a session out of hospital in his consulting room, he will telephone the ward with the time of departure, or if he is really worried he will order a taxi to take the patient back to the hospital. These arrangements are necessary with psychotic patients because any feelings of unreality can quickly lead to confusion and consequent errors in the bus or train boarded. Ward staff can come to know their patients well and can track their feelings at a surprisingly close level. Everyone benefits when the ward feels secure; patients cooperate even when very ill, and their psychological progress becomes enhanced and strengthened.

Clinical supervision, reflective practice where experiences with patients are discussed, and the practice of undergoing their own Psychoanalysis are usual methods for mental health staff to ensure that they look after themselves as well as their patients even when exposed to the psychological stress of their work. Considerable strain and pressure commonly arise in daily practice, and it is very important that each staff member is helped in these ways to deal effectively with their difficult experiences. When the staff remain secure in their work they are enabled to maintain a relaxed ward ambience where the dialogue with patients remains therapeutic and continues to be beneficial to them.

Risks may be embraced, managed, or avoided. The clinical supervision, reflective practice, and staff's own psychoanalyses mentioned above are methods of embracing risk effectively; it is anticipated, and dealt with accordingly. Managing psychological risk is a major element in Psychiatric training, and the ward Psychiatrist will be very conscious of the safety and wellbeing of all his patients. He takes this responsibility in every way, psychological and physical, on behalf of the Psychoanalyst while the schizophrenic patient in therapy is on his ward.

Risk is avoided through preventive measures. Regular fire drills, precautionary fire doors, safe arrangements for keeping locked doors unlockable should opening them be necessary, and widely established and maintained alarm systems are all ways of preventing a serious fire. Securing sufficient finance for a treatment in advance of starting it is a necessary practice to avoid psychological harm occurring to a patient when she is already exposed to unsettling mental processes and would be unable to fend for herself before her treatment's conclusion. The Psychoanalyst would try to establish this for a young person; an older adult would be advised similarly.

The ward Psychiatrist is involved both in understanding the psychoanalytically treated schizophrenic patient as well as he can, and in promoting her progress while she is most in need of care and support on his ward. The more he understands of psychotic defence mechanisms and their effects on patients' behaviour, the more he can help the Psychoanalyst and his schizophrenic patient; teaching his staff makes everyone's tasks easier in seeing through disguise, defence, ulterior unconscious motives, false selves, and all the pathological psychological structures that the schizophrenic personality may adopt in trying to preserve her Self, come what may. These false roles can be extremely beguiling and convincing, and the Psychoanalyst's experience in recognising them is greatly needed. If the ward Psychiatrist is also aware of them, he is able to teach his ward staff so that that there is cohesive effort supporting the Psychoanalyst's skilled work with his schizophrenic patient.

These aspects described of an optimal psychotherapy ward represent the ideal accommodation for a schizophrenic or schizoaffective patient who is receiving psychoanalytic psychotherapy. She is like other patients in her psychological needs on the ward, but has in addition particular needs due to factors of her illness such as confusion and often great instability due to poor resources of affect regulation and ego strength, or confident assertive ability. She may be very withdrawn at times or have a low threshold for irritability and impatience. Reliable care by the staff does help through consistency, reassurance, and trust to penetrate these superficial behavioural obstacles and reach in due course the patient's internal world, which is the source of her sometimes-psychotic communications. Further work by patient-allocated staff using care plans is an excellent way of breaking down the isolation patients may unconsciously have constructed around themselves so that they grow into better relations with those around them.

Dr Robbins' seven therapeutic stages supported by the PPCC model

Dr Michael Robbins practised psychoanalytic psychotherapy on his series of 18 paranoid schizophrenic patients at the Massachusetts Mental Health Center, and his patients were accommodated on wards in the MacLean Hospital when they were too ill to travel to see him in his consulting room (Robbins, 1993). The descriptions above of the ward care of psychotic and other patients are derived from practice at the Maudsley Hospital in London; practice can vary on either side of the Atlantic, but humane care is always the best principle to follow, and this can be and is practised in the Maudsley Hospital, emulated elsewhere.

After working for some time with different schizophrenic patients, Dr Robbins observed that his psychoanalytic psychotherapeutic treatment of his paranoid schizophrenic patients followed a sequence of seven major changes in their mental functioning, consequent upon significant adjustment in their transference relationship to him (Robbins, 1993, p.259). All his paranoid schizophrenic patients followed this sequence, including those who were unsuccessful and did not complete all of the seven stages in the process of becoming differentiated and integrated, healthy individuals; mostly these patients ceased treatment at Stage 3, having followed Stages 1 and 2. The difficulty of Stage 3, when the patient must accept the views presented by the Psychoanalyst in his interpretations even when these are at odds with what she herself is used to thinking, can provide such an obstacle that the patient is unable to overcome it. These patients are less strong than those who will emerge successfully, or else are unwilling to make the necessary changes that would enable them to continue in treatment. The unsuccessful patients leave therapy at Stage 3 when they are no longer able to cooperate with the Psychoanalyst in what he is broaching with them as the way forward. Usually this relates to an aspect of reality that he is presenting to them. The patient relinquishes effort in the direction of her own salvation, and falls away from the enterprise she had embarked upon to become healed from her faulty mental structure.

The seven therapeutic stages have direct parallels to the Psychodynamic Pentapointed Cognitive Construct (PPCC) model's description of the patient's perspective (see Table 7.1). The PPCC model describes visually, in geometric diagrams, the changes that occur in a schizophrenic or schizoaffective patient's mind as she undergoes restorative psychoanalytic psychotherapy (see Figure 7.1). The patient internalises the Psychoanalyst and, after a considerable period of years of work with him, becomes able to integrate in Time, Place, and Person as a discrete individual who can contain (three-dimensionally in the PPCC) the entirety of her life's past experiences without these provoking psychosis within her mind. She then is able to function effectively and autonomously, mixing increasingly well with other people and enabling herself to "rub off the remaining corners" of anxiety, irritability, anger, or shyness that may remain in her personality as residues from her years of illness and unhappiness. She will continue to gain strength and maturity for the rest of her life, in company with other people. Clear elucidation of the PPCC model is to be found in "The Psychiatry of Resolving Schizophrenia Psychoanalytically: How visualising the therapeutic process can assist success" (Steggles, 2019).

The two processes, the therapeutic process observed by the clinician, Dr Robbins (the seven therapeutic stages), and the process of healthy development of the patient's mind (the sequence of changes illustrated by the PPCC model) mirror each other (see Table 7.1). The PPCC model, a visual sequence of geometric shapes (see Figure 7.1), can, equally, be verbalised, and some overlap inevitably occurs between gradually succeeding stages.

The first stage is "protopathic symbiosis", or "parasitism" as Dr Robbins describes it, where the schizophrenic patient exists within the limits of her psychotic mind and relates to the Psychoanalyst on this basis, not fully comprehending what he says to her and unable to respond very constructively to him. She is dependent upon him for their

Table 7.1 Stages in the psychological resolution of schizophrenia

Stages of Psychological Therapy of Schizophrenia: Dr. Michael Robbins	PPCC Model of patient's mind: Dr. Gillian Steggles	Stages in the patient's experience
1. Protopathosymbiosis (parasitism): patient's identity is invested in her psychotic state.	Patient is unable to function Healthily using her Impoverished representational world.	Patient feels alienated in her environmental world, suffering from painful schizophrenic confusion.
2. Engagement: patient's sense of individuality is threatened.	Patient unconsciously includes analyst in her representational world.	Patient attempts to engage with analyst: she may be well-defended.
3. Pathosymbiosis: may lead to collusion and Stage 3b: Therapeutic Stalemate.	Patient's 'blocked' schizophrenic mindset may prevent mindful interaction with analyst.	Tendency towards comfortable (but false) assumptions with analyst: reality cannot be contemplated.
4. Disengagement from pathological symbiotic collusion.	Patient succeeds in rejecting her previous maladaptive relationships and unhealthy engagements in her representational world.	Patient works at reviewing her relationships and contemplating reality.
5. More normal symbiosis: growth-promoting.	Patient is awakened to the reality of her life in all its (painful) aspects of Time, Place and Person in context.	Patient is able to address reality with her analyst; she suffers painful experience of herself; she begins to understand her conflicts; she absorbs good feelings from the analyst; she begins to experience her own self-identity positively.
6. Psychic differentiation and integration.	Patient evolves into a discrete, integrated individual.	Patient can contain her own emerging integrated mental life successfully as a discrete individual, relating well to the analyst and individuating from him. Patient evolves into her own independent autonomy.
7. Therapeutic Termination.	Patient's mind is self-sufficient.	Patient leaves therapy with her difficulties resolved.

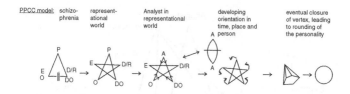

Figure 7.1 The overall sequence of changes in the mind of a schizophrenic or schizoaffective patient during psychoanalytic
psychotherapeutic resolution of the illness according to
the PPCC model.

Source: Reproduced with permission from BMJ Publishing Group Ltd. © BMJ
2017.

relationship's existence, and contributes little to its maintenance. All
she can do is to attend her sessions daily, and to sustain her responsiveness to him as well as she is able, within her limitations. Her identity
is invested in her psychotic state. Dr Robbins is saying that when the
patient is in this state, at the start of her treatment, she cannot initiate
any sensible or helpful or meaningful conversation with her Psychoanalyst. The PPCC's initial structure (see Figures 7.2 and 7.3) shows that
the patient's unpleasant, perhaps threatening representational world is
perhaps a large part of the origin of this debilitating state of mind,
within which the patient has become unable to draw enough impetus
to interact constructively with the environments around herself. The
patient therefore may feel alienated in her environments, and hence
confused and full of pain.

If the patient is able to tolerate this painful and confusing stage, she
is faced with addressing the next stage of treatment. In Stage 2, she
has to engage with the Psychoanalyst and not simply remain passively
in his company for the therapeutic hour. Her individuality, to her, is
threatened by having to accept his statements, whether about herself or
as general points about reality, and adopt these for herself: truths that
are about realities which she must endorse and use as part of herself.
The Psychoanalyst's opinions might be unpleasant to her; they may
feel threatening in some way; she may initially even feel that they are
untrue, and she may feel miserable in accepting them. However, she
has to internalise them and adopt them as her own beliefs; she may
actually not be able to understand them cognitively, and thus accepts
them on trust. These ideas may contradict what she has been brought up

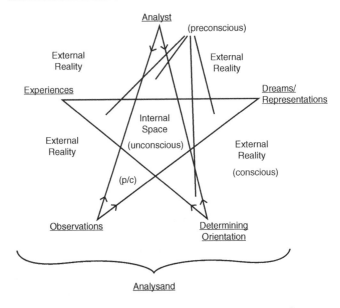

Figure 7.2 The Psychodynamic Pentapointed Cognitive Construct (PPCC) in the paranoid-schizoid position.

Source: Reproduced with permission from BMJ Publishing Group Ltd. © BMJ 2017.

with, in her family, and in thinking them she may be flying in the face of a decades-old existence, learning a different system of norms and principles. She may be aware that she is rejecting family relationships with those aged or respected individuals in her family whom she may have loved. At the time of therapy, this may seem very difficult, but trust ensures that all the good in the good members of her family from long ago is preserved: the good is retained, and sometimes the terrible faults in her family which are truly terrible but which have been hidden from her become evident. Her Psychoanalyst is her best friend in separating her from destructive ways of thinking in her family. This is why her family therapy, organised by her Psychoanalyst in liaison with her ward Psychiatrist, is so complex, and why the ward Psychiatrist and his ward staff really must trust and support the Psychoanalyst as he tries to fend off the family's damaging influence on his patient. The family

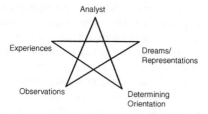

<u>Psychoanalyst</u>
Directs therapeutic activities towards resolving analysand's problems

<u>Experiences</u>
Childhood trauma
Neglect by mother
Inadequate nourishment
Exposure to danger by mother and by self
Insensitivity and emotional unavailability of father
Exposure to severe isolation abroad when only a child
Family pride in equating strength and maturity with masculinity and expectation of
suppression of emotion

<u>Dreams/Representations</u>
Mentally unstable mother
Emotionally absent father
'Macho' brothers, one of whom she was fond of, but one who queried her need for
hospitalization
Conveyed impression of self as a person of indeterminate gender, and believed that she, like
all girls, was a castrated male.
Dream: of a great family dining-room in a cylindrical 8-storey building containing
dangerously floating tables and chairs which could be injurious. A clown caused the death of
her sister.

<u>Observations</u> (non-psychotic thoughts)
Patient was "getting a few crumbs"
"I really think I am alive, and if I think about it I get so sad and I get really angry".

<u>Determining Orientation</u> (psychosis and disturbed behaviour)
Tried to be inconspicuous and hide herself from her mother, including a badly cut finger.
Tried to run away from home to skid row areas of cities, where her low self-esteem allowed
men to abuse her sexually in exchange for food and a place to sleep.

Figure 7.3 An example of the PPCC representational world, from one
of Dr Robbins' patients.

members are not at fault unless they fail to respect the Psychoanalyst's work with their compromised relative. The patient's sense of individuality has been threatened by them, often unconsciously and therefore unawares, throughout her lifetime with them, and her Psychoanalyst tries hard to restore it within her family therapy, while continuing his work with her in her individual psychoanalytic psychotherapy.

The PPCC model at Stage 2 illustrates the assumption by the Psychoanalyst of his position at the top of the model, and influential within his patient's mind. As a good internal object within her, he is able to strengthen her efforts on her own behalf, and in therapeutic conversation to guide her thinking into an increasing awareness of reality. The patient, on her part, will be making increasing efforts to engage with him in spite of perhaps quite strong family ties.

Stage 3 of the psychoanalytic psychotherapy of schizophrenia involves the possibility of the therapy terminating prematurely. The pathological nature of the therapeutic relationship that is due to the patient's own psychological restrictions may have subliminal or unintended benefits for the Psychoanalyst. He may simply unconsciously enjoy the patient's dependence on him. If he is unwilling or unable to assert truth and reality to his patient, the patient may slowly decline in her contributions to the treatment, her interest in the Psychoanalyst's words and her treatment will cease, and the therapy will grind to a halt. This would be the end of her treatment due to therapeutic stalemate. The PPCC model for schizophrenia (Figure 7.4) shows that the patient's mind is blocked internally, and is unable to permit insightful, properly functioning interaction with the Psychoanalyst, who may or may not be engaging in collusion with the patient; but

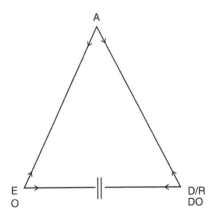

Figure 7.4 The PPCC in schizophrenia.

Source: Reproduced with permission from BMJ Publishing Group Ltd. © BMJ 2017.

communication between the therapeutic dyad fails either way, and the patient's progress will stall. This will be a tremendous loss for the patient; she, and often her family also, will have invested greatly in her therapy, so to lose its proffered opportunity for her to gain her health is to lose her once in a lifetime chance for her future. Her Psychoanalyst will not give up lightly, but if he feels he really cannot help her to make further progress he must be honest and broach this reality to her.

But Stage 4 offers the opposite choice to the patient. She becomes able to disengage not from the Psychoanalyst but from the pathological symbiotic collusion that threatened the therapeutic dyad due to the patient's adherence to her past values. To adopt Stage 4 is real progress for the patient. She has succeeded in rejecting her previous maladaptive relationships and unhealthy engagements in her representational world; she can now work at reviewing her relationships and contemplating the realities presented to her by her Psychoanalyst. She needs to see him no longer as her sole supplier of resilience, resourcefulness, and strength, but rather to regard herself as an independent agent, and responsible for herself. The PPCC model shows the patient alternating healthily between the paranoid-schizoid and depressive positions, with the Psychoanalyst remaining in his influential position at the top of both structures. This stage requires motivation in the patient, with a real effort towards reviewing herself in relation to the environment around herself, including especially observing objectively her family and unhealthy ties to her deficient representational world.

Stage 5 consists of a more symbiotic, growth-promoting relationship between the Psychoanalyst and his patient. Having detached from her original restricting representational world, the patient is awakened to the reality of her life in all its painful aspects. The pain is the result of seeing much more clearly how past circumstances and situations contributed to her mental deficits, and that she must now leave all of these behind if she is to become truly herself. She can now adjust to and relate to her past events and experiences in terms of Time, Place, and Person so that they no longer tend to cause her confusion, unhappiness, and psychotic illness. This is illustrated by the PPCC model becoming three-dimensional and containing all her past experiences and memories in a five-sided pyramid, and the patient adding constructively to these as the model moves forwards in time. In clinical terms, the patient is able now to address reality with her Psychoanalyst. She suffers painfully upon learning that she is who she is, faults and all. She can now see, upon looking back at her past, what her own contributions to her illness have been; if she had responded differently to previous situations and circumstances then perhaps she might have been able to process them differently and caused them to have a different effect upon her, the same effect on her as she now remembers them. As it is, she can now look back upon them quite harmlessly and experience no drive towards psychosis from them. Absorbing good feelings from her Psychoanalyst helps the patient tremendously to progress from day to day as she relives her memories differently: previously very painfully but now somewhat philosophically. In doing so, she begins to experience herself as a discrete person, with her own identity and in a positive light.

When psychic differentiation and integration come about in the patient she has reached Stage 6. She has learned to rely upon herself in bad times as well as good times, and to hold her own opinions based on reality and solid experience. She has her own distinct personality and holds herself together, integrated and with her own identity. Unlike her early family influences, the people she now spends time with do not cast expectations upon her that warp and distort her view of herself. She probably has little exchange with her family by now, and her mind and her representational world are peopled by individuals who recognise and accept her as she sees herself, not seeing her through an overwhelming and mistaken lens. Among similarly evolved, integrated individuals like her friends, the patient can contain her own emerging integrated mental life successfully, relating well to her Psychoanalyst and differentiating from him. The patient individuates and evolves into her own independent autonomy. The PPCC model's overall sequence shows all of this in its representation of her as a sphere, a solid individual with "all her corners rubbed off" and able to move smoothly in her life without crises, difficulties or obstructions any more than the usual untoward events that are to be expected.

Therapeutic termination is the final stage, at Stage 7. The patient is able to use her mind to help herself through life's difficulties when these occur. She is self-sufficient and can determine her own goals and progress, and leaves therapy in a healed state with only residual effects of her illness requiring monitoring and sufficient effort to let her enjoy her new-found health.

Staging the psychoanalytic psychotherapy of schizophrenic patients is helpful because it allows closer comparison between different patients undergoing the same treatment than if comparison remained based only on overall progress. The seven stages relate to the changing relationship of the patient to her therapist (see Table 7.1). The PPCC's evaluation of these differing relationship types describes verbally the changes in the patient's mind at each stage, in parallel and overall (see Table 7.1). Diagrammatically the PPCC describes the overall process, although not diagrams on a 1:1 basis with the seven stages (see Figure 7.1). Changes in the patient's mind affected by schizophrenia are elucidated in these ways, and it is helpful to know how the mechanism of therapy of schizophrenia brings about its results.

The Psychoanalyst practising psychoanalytic psychotherapy with a schizophrenic patient adopts and practises his own psychoanalytic technique, greatly adapted as patient-centred therapy. Keeping his eye on the progress of his patient, through Dr Robbins' stages or according to the authority he follows, he will observe features of schizophrenia identified many years ago by his forebears, commonly in Britain of the Kleinian School. When his patient has made good progress and no longer manifests frank symptoms but is able to internalise what he says to her and reflect on her own internal processes, he may identify aspects of her mind now in common with less ill patients studied by psychoanalytic authorities, perhaps again from the Kleinian School.

Dr Robbins maintained that he did not follow any one school of Psychoanalysis, but adopted an eclectic approach useful to his own very much patient-centred psychoanalytic technique that he used on his paranoid schizophrenic patients. With this technique he achieved good results, one-third of his 18 patients achieving "a very successful outcome", and a further three patients achieving "a positive result".

Four therapeutically accessible systems from Dr Robbins' hierarchy of eight systems

Dr Robbins did, however, develop his own Theory of Mind, to which he adhered in the management of his patients. This was his Hierarchy of eight Systems for schizophrenia (Robbins, 1993, p.33), a concept developed from John Gedo's work that advocated the concept of Hierarchical Systems as having potential in the development of psychoanalytic theory (Gedo, 1979, 1984, 1986, 1988). Each system is neither reducible to lower systems nor predictable from them: molecular biology, neurobiology, neurochemistry, Psychoanalysis, interpersonal psychology, family systems, sociology, and cultural anthropology.

From this Hierarchy, four Systems may be developed as a hierarchy of the care required for patients, which can be explained by evidence for the pathological processes understood to be causing schizophrenia:

i At the neurophysiological-pharmacological level, it is known that excess dopamine is secreted in the brain in schizophrenia, and that this is closely related to schizophrenic symptoms. Antipsychotic medications suppress the excessive production of dopamine, leading to abatement of the psychotic symptoms.

ii The psychological symptoms of schizophrenia are tackled most effectively using psychoanalytic psychotherapy. The Psychiatry-trained Psychoanalyst sees his patient up to five times per week in his consulting-room, or in hospital if she is too ill to travel to see him. Over time, she gains insight into her condition and learns to function despite difficulties that may remain from her past pain. Her relief at understanding what used to prevent her living normally gives her inspiration to persevere, and she takes her opportunity at living her future life.

iii Family therapy enables her family to catch up with her progress. They may co-operate in doing this, but resentment and even anger may surface if their habitual attitudes towards her are challenged by the Psychoanalyst and another staff member in the family therapy group. The therapists try to inform and guide the family into kinder and more respectful ways of relating to her, now that she can speak for herself and has her own ideas about how she wishes to be understood.

iv She may decide to leave her family and set out to find her own community, but on the best terms possible.

v She may develop needs for social help as she moves forward into the community where she hopes to live in future. If these are met, her own initiative is likely to see her through the early stages of her rehabilitation, ready and keen to make the most of her new opportunities. Keeping in touch with the hospital to begin with gives her confidence to do so, until her need for her carers' help diminishes.

This hierarchy of four therapeutic Systems attends to all the levels at which schizophrenic illness impinges on the patient's life. Some levels overlap in time as they are applied, such as medication provision benefiting the patient during her psychoanalytic psychotherapy and family therapy. The hospital and the Psychoanalyst's consulting-room not far away provide the basis for this comprehensive approach to enabling the patient to address and fully overcome the illness' effects on her. Allowing her to see for herself how she can resolve its influence over her is the treatment that enables her to treat herself, long after she no longer sees her doctors, the therapeutic gift that goes on giving.

References

Gedo, J (1979). *Beyond Interpretation*. New York: International Universities Press.

Gedo, J (1984). *Psychoanalysis and its Discontents*. New York: Guilford Press.

Gedo, J (1986). *Conceptual Issues in Psychoanalysis*. Hillsdale, NJ: Analytic Press.

Gedo, J (1988). *The Mind in Disorder*. Hillsdale, NJ: Analytic Press.

Robbins, M (1993). *Experiences of Schizophrenia: An Integration of the Personal, Scientific and Therapeutic*. New York: Guilford Press.

Steggles, G (2019). The Psychiatry of Resolving Schizophrenia Psychoanalytically: How Visualizing the Therapeutic Process Can Assist Success. UK: Free Association Books.

Chapter 8

Difficulties encountered during psychoanalytic psychotherapy and overcoming them

Schizophrenic illness affects the whole of the patient's mind; it prevents normal thinking until medication has been taken by the patient, and sometimes this state persists. The patient's mind is preserved as energetically as possible by staff early in the illness through conversation with her and reassurance; the duration of untreated psychosis is kept to an absolute minimum. If she has shown responsiveness and accessibility, and has demonstrated premorbid application and effort and intelligent efforts to progress in her life then she may be considered to have good potential in psychoanalytic psychotherapy. She may be given a trial period of six months or so in treatment to assess how she responds, with a view to full treatment.

The illness tends to involve complicated and difficult-to-manage psychological phenomena that may also be seen in other mental conditions. For example, the false self that some schizophrenic patients disclose, in the nature of Donald Winnicott's concept of problematic inauthenticity (Winnicott, 1965a) that he saw as a core problem, can create major difficulty for the Psychoanalyst, who does not then know who he is working with. But with experience, he learns to recognise these difficulties and find his way forward.

Psychotic defences

Psychotic defences have been seen (in Chapters 3 and 6) to create confusion regarding the patient within their family and initially also for therapeutic staff caring for her. These defences interfere with mentalisation and prevent clear communication also between the therapeutic dyad, the Psychoanalyst, and the analysand (the patient). Non-psychotic or neurotic defences are particularly commonly encountered

DOI: 10.4324/9781003433507-12

in family therapy, where each family member tries hard to defend themselves and justify their views when the actual dynamics affecting the patient are brought to their notice. For example, the mother of Dr Robbins' patient Sara exhibited psychotic defences when Sara and staff tried to engage with her:

> Sara tried to talk to her mother about her feelings of having been neglected, and she told me that in response her mother became enraged, called Sara a bitch, threw an ashtray against the wall, and resisted efforts of staff to calm her. Our responses to her story were curiously congruent; I wondered if Sara had imagined all this (that her mother was actually normal) and Sara herself did not find anything [un]remarkable about her description of her mother's behaviour. Interestingly, her mother's crazy behaviour was subsequently confirmed in its particulars by a staff member who had been present.
>
> (Robbins, 2012, p.586)
> (Reprinted with permission of Dr Michael
> Robbins and Guilford Press)

The recurring incomprehensibility of the patient, who at times may be quite inscrutable, poses real difficulty for the clinician. Dr Robbins was trained to sit with his patients while they suffered their experience of themselves in his consulting room. He had his Theory of Mind, his Hierarchical Systems Theory (see Robbins, 1993, pp. 142–4, and Chapter 7) to refer to and keep himself intact, solid, and strong, so his compassion did not lead to identification in any way with his patient. He was able to find a way through his patients' difficulties so that he could then help them to find their way out into better mental health.

His patients' deviousness, sometimes due to inauthenticity involving an unconscious false self and consequently misleading, was hard for him to withstand, as he found with Sara:

> She said, very convincingly, that she was upset because she had been untruthful with me and that she really did not hallucinate, and the stories of abuse and skid row were fabrications. She said when she was in London and had wanted attention and sympathy she went to a restaurant and convinced the waiter that she was a bereaved widow revisiting the scene of her marriage. I felt shocked and a bit sick to my stomach and I wondered aloud whether I could trust my senses about what was real. Sara tried to convince me that

she was telling me these 'truths' because our relationship was deepening and she cared, but I felt suspicious, a bit paranoid as I struggled with what was real.

(Robbins, 2012, pp.589–90)
(Reprinted with permission of Dr Michael
Robbins and Guilford Press)

These aspects of the patient make it hard for the Psychoanalyst to deliver psychoanalytic psychotherapy to her, and he has to be well aware of their possible appearance in her at all times so that he can sustain his own wellbeing. Furthermore, self-harming is often linked to deviousness in concealing her aggression against herself; this can be shocking and also emotionally upsetting. Dr Robbins was affected in this way by his concern for her, but still tried to allow his patient to realise, herself, what she had done to herself so unnecessarily. Freedom to explore their own experiences as themselves was key to his therapeutic approach to his patients.

Understanding schizophrenia is difficult because the illness is highly complex and affects the patient in at least the four different specified strata among Dr Robbins' Hierarchy of eight Systems. There is no doubt that there is excess dopamine in some nerve tracts such as the mesolimbic tract in the brains of schizophrenic patients. Psychoanalysis itself does not have the tools to understand this or discuss it, but produces understanding through its own psychotherapeutic application. Neuroscientific thinking and psychoanalytic therapy together in themselves provide possibilities for understanding and effective treatment. As referred to above, the Hierarchy of Systems advocated by Dr Michael Robbins does present a method and a form of understanding through which different aspects of schizophrenic illness' effects on the patient's mind may be tackled.

Mentalising, its impedence, and therapy

Schizophrenia appears to involve impairment in mentalising ability, the ability to cogitate and actively understand other minds. This, in turn, may be due to psychotic defence mechanisms, as Freud concluded from his study of the highly intelligent Judge Schreber's paranoid and hypochondriac delusions (Freud, 1911) which interfered with his working life and precipitated his admission to several mental asylums; or to neurocognitive failure manifesting as structurally based deficits in processing or mentalising. This point supports Karl Jaspers' important distinction, made in 1913, between personality development and process or endogenous schizophrenia (Jaspers, 1913).

The role of the Psychoanalyst's clinical skills is to identify and interpret to the patient aspects of her life which she has brought to him, so that she can understand them better, learn from them, and then use her new understanding accordingly. Endogenously incapacitated schizophrenic patients who suffer from compromised neurological functioning can find their limitations will not allow them to make use of psychoanalytic sessions. The stresses of psychoanalytic psychotherapy, utilising the Psychoanalyst's interpretations in internal reflection, are best borne by cognitively intense effort, combined with the personal qualities active in the transference of patience, tolerance, forgiveness, curiosity, and determination needed to persevere with the therapy. It is the task of the Psychoanalyst to alleviate functional psychological block; but he can do nothing about structural block. The therapist of schizophrenic patients will flexibly adjust his clinical technique as the patient's mind increasingly becomes more receptive under his influence, as part of the changing transference relationship. If a patient is restricted even in a positive transference from utilising the interpretations successfully, through structural block or another cause, the therapy will reach an impasse after such benefit as she has managed to glean, and can go no further.

Overcoming difficulties

The Psychoanalyst overcomes such difficulties as he encounters when he psychoanalyses his schizophrenic patient through his clinical skills. With experience, he recognises tendencies common in schizophrenia that are painful to observe and hard to remedy. His patient's pain as she is subjected to her mental states is difficult for the Psychoanalyst to alleviate; early on, he can only comment empathically and sit and await his perception of meaning as it emerges from her in due course. Then he can support or enlighten what she says. Deducing meaning from confused, disconnected abstractions and bizarre behaviour is very difficult (see Chapters 3 and 6), and at these times the Psychoanalyst can only wait until psychotic experience no longer prevents the patient from communicating meaningfully with him; Psychoanalysts do not often try to communicate with their schizophrenic patients "on the psychotic wavelength" (Lucas, 2009), though some may wish to try to open this channel to their patients.

The clinician's skills improve with time as he learns about his patient, and as he treats further patients and recognises features common to them; Dr Robbins eventually recognised aspects of his relationships with all the patients he treated that these had in common, sufficiently so that he was able to establish seven therapeutic Stages that they all reached between the start and the successful ending of their treatment, or so far as they progressed with him. Confidence and courage are always valued in a Psychoanalyst's working experience; and useful default skills that can be picked up are especially applicable to complex cases where the ongoing processes at any one moment are difficult to define: remaining silent, if the Psychoanalyst is unsure; echoing what has just been said, to encourage the patient; and offering a brief resume of the session so far, if the Psychoanalyst feels the patient has lost track of the flow of meaning between themselves. These are examples of filling time during which the patient's state of mind may become clearer. Bringing his patient's responses to his Supervisor is another good way to help the Psychoanalyst question or confirm his initial views when he feels unsure of a clinical point. Recurring incomprehensibility in his patient can be very difficult to tolerate long term. Time goes by, and is precious to everyone; yet one of Dr Robbins' patients, Sara, stated to him, once she had recovered, that it was his sitting with her hour after hour when she was at her most ill that she remembers above almost all other aspects of her therapy.

The Psychoanalyst's powers of observation are one of his own best friends. Further to observations, reflection upon them in connection with time, previously remarked findings, and in connection with other patients, may reveal conclusions which he can use on future occasions in his patient's therapy. He may begin to observe her traits, her habits, and her tendencies, and he may become able to predict her responses to what he says to her. She will at the same time be beginning, unconsciously to start with, to feel the improvement in her communication with him. She may react to this, perhaps with anxiety, or nonchalance, or relief; through his observations, he will be able to guide her into discovery of her own potential in using this strengthened relationship. He can refer to her recent responses and ask her about them; in recognising these as the improvements in her that they represent, she may well feel encouraged. Remaining alert and observing acutely can make the Psychoanalyst's task easier, being quicker to pick up on his patient's progress. Kindness of approach and consistency of openness in the Psychoanalyst remain one of the surest foundations of a patient's progress when she has many difficulties; she will respond to his observations and interpretations much more surely and hopefully when he has become fully accessible to her through his available openness towards her.

The Psychoanalyst's stance towards his patient is necessarily consistent, even when her behaviour has been unpredictable and her mental state less than easy to follow. If she is projecting into him aggressive feelings, or suffering from envy or feels persecuted by him, it may be hard for him to continue to tolerate these in her while she rages and articulates her pain. He will be used to patients expressing hostility towards him; but tolerating this as far as possible, and interpreting what he can, will allow her the experience of exploring her anger safely. His patience with her is his best approach, assisted by active interpretations which make her think about her feelings and, if he is able, help her seek explanations for them as to their source. Her desire to be well will be driving her to try her hardest to comply with the analysis' requirements, and she will have been given the chance of her therapy on the grounds of her accessibility and responsiveness.

His Theory of Mind will provide the foundation of the Psychoanalyst's choice of responses to his patients. For much of the time, his approach to his schizophrenic patients will be patient-centred, especially at the start of their therapy with him. Using this approach, he will come to learn their traits and foibles and tendencies to respond to similar remarks made by him in their own way that becomes familiar. Once their illness' symptoms have been resolved or at least become known to him in a more manageable way than at first, he may recognise in his patients more generally applicable psychological behaviour. Many Psychoanalysts in the UK belong to the Kleinian School, and this provides a sound basis for psychoanalytic practice. Having grown more integrated and internally aware, a schizophrenic patient is likely still to suffer aspects of her illness which may be observed by the Psychoanalyst; but he is then able to refer to the observations of the Kleinian School Psychoanalysts who followed Klein, and her own work, and identify in his patient what they discovered and wrote about. His patient will manifest projective identification, split, and defend herself vigorously from painful ideas that he may try to persuade her to discuss about her own life. She will have a lot of anxiety, paranoid and manic and, perhaps, depressive too if schizoaffective, since schizoid patients suffer quite severely from anxieties of different kinds on a continuous basis. Bion's substantial contributions will provide the

Psychoanalyst of schizophrenic patients with many examples of the strange ways the patient's mind differs from non-psychotic minds. That Rosenfeld's patient Mildred was alleviated completely of her schizophrenia by him should give the Psychoanalyst some hope and belief, along with Dr Robbins' patients and Dr Steggles' research patient. A schizophrenic patient's language can be extremely strange, such as in one of Bion's patients, thinking that a gramophone is watching her. As he interprets, it is as if a part of her mind, the part that watches, has wrapped itself around the gramophone and become a "bizarre object"; then what could be more natural than that the gramophone is watching her? The strangeness of a part of her mind wrapping itself around the gramophone as a projective identification is part of the strangeness of schizophrenic mental behaviour, a development of a phenomenon identified originally by Bion's predecessors Freud and Klein. Our Psychoanalyst of schizophrenic patients can, in the Kleinian School, feel reassured by all his literary clinical colleagues, and enjoy recognising what is happening in his patient, in order to draw, in a cogent way, to her attention how her own mind may be playing tricks on her but that this is only part of her illness; and with time, as she talks more about her experiences, she is likely to become better connected with other people's minds.

Factors helpful to the patient

There are many aspects of psychoanalytic psychotherapy that can be rendered helpful for schizophrenic and schizoaffective patients. If the patient can be helped to feel warmly towards her Psychoanalyst this makes a big difference to the benefit she can derive from her sessions. She is likely to try harder to help herself if she genuinely feels benefit from her encounters with him during her sessions. It is very much to be hoped that a schizophrenic patient who can engage in a transference with her prospective Psychoanalyst has within her a genuine, feeling human being; this person grew up and developed with much difficulty in her environment but, after suffering greatly, on being given the chance to emerge out of her illness will take it and work hard to try to do so in her therapeutic alliance with her Psychoanalyst, and manifest her humanity.

The closer the offer of treatment can be made to the onset of her psychosis, once she has been assessed and definite confirmation of her willingness to work hard and persevere in the long term with her treatment has been made, the better preserved her natural personality and the accessibility of her transference are likely to be. Sometimes psychoanalytic psychotherapy has to be postponed, if there are other considerations such as another dependent family member or educational demands. Patients with a psychotic breakdown are cared for by the health system in Britain, and if they comply with treatment the system will do its best to provide effective treatments that will enable the patient to reach her functional goals. More Psychiatric Psychoanalysts are being trained who increasingly know how to relate psychoanalytically to schizophrenic patients so that, through accessing their miserable, isolated, deprived, frightened selves who have been restricted through their inexplicably pained experiences, the patients become enabled to articulate what, for them, has been the actual difficulty they have been facing as they tried to develop. A good transference can inspire a patient, once they are well into their therapy, to do really well in terms of "sorting themselves out" after leaving their early environment which created such an unpleasant representational world as they experienced early on in their life; nobody's fault can be held to account for this unpleasantness, as family life is known to be extremely difficult and stressful for parents especially, and siblings do their best to get on with each other in the circumstances. One child may seem to come off worst on a regular basis; it is important for an adult to address this so that connection can be established with the child and they learn self-expression and standing up for themselves. Assertiveness may be a potential protector from schizophrenia, which often develops after much deep-seated dysphoria and internal disquiet, withdrawal and isolation. The importance of the transference to the quality of a patient's progress is reflected in the meaningfulness to them of their learning with their Psychoanalyst; each of the two effects of the treatment enhances the other.

Countertransference, likewise, is important to the patient, for them to feel warmed from the frozen experiences they have been living through. The Psychoanalyst's professionalism and maintenance of "evenly-suspended, positive regard" may be all he does feel for his patient, but his constancy, consistent level of attention, the even tone of his voice and unarousability to anything beyond calm reassurance and encouraging interest will allow her to feel connection with him that she can express in exactly the form in which this arises in her. Having this person, her Psychoanalyst, alongside her as she increasingly tries to make sense of herself, at a deep level eventually, is the framework within which her schizophrenia really does have its best chance of being resolved. Her Psychoanalyst will himself have lived through her tussles with herself in a manner hidden from her by his calm exterior; his actual feelings he will talk through in his own self-analysis with a colleague, but his ability to understand and live through her difficulties as far as these affect him, while being for her a secure, enlightened and kindly emotionally reflecting mirror to which she can bring her experiences as she has them, is the irreplaceable resource that she can utilise to become well.

This opportunity, a truly life-saving event, being offered this treatment, needs to be made available to many more schizophrenic patients who at present wait in little hope of receiving it. Work is under way towards this aim; and it rests on clinicians who after years of professional training may take on the great challenge of studying this illness: while they preserve themselves in the best health possible in order to do so. Knowledge and experience gained will reassure everyone involved in the patients' treatment that the illness is being mastered. It is quite variable in its manifestation; which is why patient-centred therapy especially at the start of treatment is necessary. The Psychoanalyst's countertransference, his connection to his patient despite all the confusion she causes him, may hold him in courage while he does his work with her. As described, it is to be hoped that she, underneath the illness' psychotic symptoms, is a nice and decent human being who essentially validates in terms of human generosity and kindly substance all his efforts with her. She may have become sharp and aggressive because of the years of frustration and difficulty she has lived through with her illness. But in a successful Psychoanalysis, she will be able to realise these aspects of herself, which her Psychoanalyst's consistency and the sufficiency of his countertransference to her can bring out to inspection, and then leave her human self, nearly dead but surviving underneath in her soul, to emerge and flourish instead of her illness. The schizophrenic patient is greatly helped in this by knowledge from early in her life, if she can be helped to remember a happy early time before her symptoms began to develop. If she can be reminded of herself as a good and nice and quite content person early in her life by her Psychoanalyst, they can both work on the idea "so what became different between then and now?". His own countertransference, apart from his training, will help him in this.

The patient's narrative provides the material of the analysis; her Psychoanalyst listens carefully, at all times letting her express what she can. Her ability to do this improves as she begins to recover. If he takes care to frame his interpretations always in a kindly way, and has an ability himself, if a rebuke is necessary, to do this in a way which affects her in the way intended but does not overwhelm her, then she will make good strides forward in learning to articulate her narrative. It is this, her narrative, which progresses through her treatment, containing all the incidents of her learning, her mistakes, and her confusions and upsets, which her Psychoanalyst observes from his therapeutic perspective. If he pursues his principle of being kind to her, despite these difficulties of hers described above which have emerged because of the stress and unpleasantness of being ill with her illness, she will be less afraid to bring to him her issues; she can only become well if she airs these issues with him; if he is approachable through good transference and good countertransference then the worst aspects of her entire illness will emerge. This was Freud's theory; and he almost certainly never envisaged what might be possible in 2023. But he was proud of every step his brainchild of Psychoanalysis took in becoming a useful treatment. In "On the History of the Psycho-Analytic Movement" he wrote:

> [Bleuler] showed that light could be thrown on a large number of purely psychiatric cases by adducing the same processes as have been recognised through psycho-analysis to obtain in dreams and neuroses (Freudian mechanisms); and Jung [in "The Psychology of Dementia Praecox", in 1907] successfully applied the analytic method of interpretation to the most alien and obscure phenomena of dementia praecox [schizophrenia], so that their sources in the life-history and interests of the patient came clearly to light. After this it was impossible for psychiatrists to ignore psycho-analysis any longer. Bleuler's great work on schizophrenia ["Dementia Praecox, or the Group of Schizophrenias"] (1911), in which the psycho-analytic point of view was placed on an equal footing with the clinical systematic one, completed this success.
>
> (Freud, 1915b, p.28)

In 2023, Psychiatric and Psychoanalytic knowledge, when combined, relate as equivalent partners in understanding schizophrenia when previously, in Freud's day, they saw schizophrenia from different, earnestly adhered-to viewpoints which were seen as challengingly rivalrous at best, and incompatible at worst; schizophrenia's study was still in its early stages. The two viewpoints are now seen constructively as each contributing essential information about the illness. Patients benefit enormously from the two professions' concerted efforts to help them understand themselves, assisted both by helpful medications which tackle brain tissue dysfunction and by gently interceding, exploratory, and explanatory therapeutic interpretations by an approachable Psychoanalyst that enable the patient to recognise and understand for herself her own life.

The schizophrenic patient's Psychoanalyst remains calm when aroused affect becomes apparent in her during a session. He will do his best to contain her, and reaffirm that she try to describe to him exactly what is going on for her and tell him about it, for understanding her accessed emotion is how her deep disturbance will eventually be calmed. In Britain, a lower level of arousal is permitted in treatment than in other countries; if the patient becomes emotionally aroused or distracted then she should be sent back to hospital in a taxi and visited by the Psychoanalyst there; her usual journey back would not be safe in that condition. Aroused feelings are capably worked through with the ward staff, and can be discussed with the Psychoanalyst in a calm way during subsequent sessions. No manifestations of any kind of violent behaviour are tolerated in British hospitals without being addressed with the patient; talking and reasoning are always the first approach, with physical measures resorted to only if the patient is completely out of touch with the nursing staff. An injection of a benzodiazepine or a major tranquilliser may have to be given to restore calm in the patient; no one likes this having to be done if words or oral administration prove ineffective. A lot of psychotherapy in the ward groups and with nurse therapists there has to be done before attendance at her sessions can be resumed. All this can be done with kindness, however; many patients will not forget either their management nor the kindness.

The Psychoanalyst needs to maintain strict boundaries in his practice. Timing; strict boundaries of respect for him and for the treatment; clear arrangements for funding the treatment; whether or not the patient is given alternative ways of contacting him out of hours, all need to be crystal clear to the patient. This helps her avoid anxiety concerning them. She has more than enough anxiety to manage in her own life, and simple routines help her to concentrate on herself.

The patient is helped to proceed with tackling her illness if external reality, which she may have had difficulties in relating to, is represented as being less fearful and less difficult to address than she had earlier found. When she is still without clear ego boundaries or is still unclear how she feels she may have strange ideas about the world; unrealistic anxieties and attitudes may prevail, and she may prefer to ignore it. On growing stronger, her Psychoanalyst's capable, encouraging ideas about it may help her to integrate into the world. If the possibility of any specific danger is anticipated, it is important that simple, clear advice is presented to her in order to enable her to avoid it; both her strange ideas (possibly due to family contacts) and poor mentalising ability may otherwise seriously expose her to it.

Curiosity can be a great stimulus and contribution to an analysis that can help the Psychoanalyst introduce an idea to the patient. It can usher in a fresh approach if a problem has been examined thoroughly by both parties, thought about, and explored in recent sessions, but still remains unresolved. The patient may be interested, especially if the transference is good, in what the Psychoanalyst produces, if he announces that he "is curious". It is, after all, about her; with a will they may both consider and re-examine together this topic. She will feel grateful for this bond of a shared activity that can enlighten her experience of her therapy.

Patients feel secure in their Psychoanalysis with a consistent, patient, warm Psychoanalyst; this applies to schizophrenic and schizoaffective patients as much as to patients with other problems. Even in the early stages of their treatment, perhaps especially so, they benefit from this security. The Psychoanalysis is hard work for both of the therapeutic pair, but concentrating on its continuity and the long view is how it will succeed.

References

Freud, S (1911). Psycho-analytical notes on an autobiographical account of a case of paranoia (Dementia Paranoides). In: *The Standard Edition of the Complete Psychological Works of Sigmund Freud*, Ed. Strachey, J. Vol. XII, pp.3–82. London: Vintage (2001).

Freud, S (1915b). On the history of the psycho-analytic movement. In: *The Standard Edition of the Complete Psychological Works of Sigmund Freud*, Ed. Strachey, J. Vol. XIV, p.28. London: Vintage (2001).

Jaspers, K (1913). *Allgemeine Psychopathologie*. Springer: Berlin. *General Psychopathology*, 7th Edn. Transl. Hoenig, J; Hamilton, M. Manchester: Manchester University Press (1959).

Lucas, R (2009). *The Psychotic Wavelength*. London and New York: Routledge.

Robbins, M (1993). *Experiences of Schizophrenia: An Integration of the Personal, Scientific and Therapeutic.* New York: Guilford Press.

Robbins, M (2012). The successful psychoanalytic therapy of a schizophrenic woman. *Psychodynamic Psychiatry*, 40(4):575–608. Reproduced with permission of Dr Michael Robbins and Guilford Press.

Winnicott, D (1965a). Ego distortion in terms of true and false self. In: *The Maturational Process and the Facilitating Environment*, Ed. Winnicott, D. pp.140–52. New York: International Universities Press.

Chapter 9

Maintaining psychological wellbeing during the treatment process

Underpinning the whole psychoanalytic psychotherapy treatment is the Psychoanalyst's own health. The Psychoanalyst's health is his most precious possession. Like most others, he will benefit from a circle of contacts: loved ones, friends, and colleagues. His is a special case regarding support, however, since those working with patients' mental health are considered to be exposed to risk but to benefit so much from their own personal Psychoanalysis that in many centres this is a requirement. It is important that he finds a colleague who can review his health for him on a regular basis, so that he does not become isolated in his own mind or feel disconnected from everyday life due to working hard with his patients (Robbins, 1993). His professional colleagues, societies, institutes, and academic conferences will all provide for him means of associating and engaging creatively outside his working hours. Fresh ideas and stimulation with friends as well will allow him to see his patients from a healthy, human perspective as well as from an academic, theoretical stance that his training will have endowed him with.

The human touch

Patients respond well to 'the human touch' in environments as unusual for them, and as strict, as the psychoanalytic setting. Occasional laughter, if it happens, certainly strengthens the bond between Psychoanalyst and patient if the analysis reaches a point where the patient is no longer deeply immersed in despair or anxiety. Laughter will be remembered (Argyle, 1987; Huppert et al, 2005), and perhaps colour the patient's experience of her treatment in a very positive light; it will only happen if the Psychoanalyst is in a good state of mental health and enjoying his

DOI: 10.4324/9781003433507-13

work. Psychoanalysis is extremely hard, and commonly very difficult work, so the Psychoanalyst does very well if he continues strongly in good health; and this he will be communicating to his patient so that she benefits as well. It comes from the Psychoanalyst taking real care of himself, so that he can take care of his patients; this effort will help him or her to remain sufficiently tough to fulfil his or her roles well.

The patient's health, being the material managed by the therapy, is what occupies the Psychoanalyst's and the hospital staff's attention, receiving a great deal of work from them all. The patient's attention is focused on it as well, but it is often also true that on the psychotherapy ward the staff receive a lot of affection from the patients. When psychotherapy is not the ward's approach this tends to be less true, and the ward is not such a happy place. But psychotherapy brings with it good feeling, always from the staff but also to a considerable extent from the patients, who become aware during their stay on it of their relationships within that community, among patients and staff alike. They realise how grateful they are to the staff members, and share their feelings about it. Staff training will have been undergone, but personal contributions by everybody give tremendous hope to the patients, most of whom have left very painful scenes behind in order to learn better how to understand themselves and live their lives.

Strong bonds on the ward provide an excellent anchor for the schizophrenic or schizoaffective patient while she attends her psychoanalytic psychotherapeutic session with her Psychoanalyst. She has been given every chance to work out how she can endure better or increasingly gain insights into challenging her thinking and responses due to her illness. Does she have to feel this? Can she find a better way of managing her reactions so that they become less painful? The more she is encouraged to ask herself questions, supported while she does this perhaps by a nurse therapist with a care plan on the ward, the better use she can make of her sessions with her Psychoanalyst. He will also be listening to how she is progressing, and asking her his own questions when she grows quiet or if what she says is not quite clear – to clarify her to herself as much as to him. It is the patient's own understanding of herself which is the bottom line in mental health therapy; every aspect of therapy is focused on enabling her to manage her own life. The difficulties that schizophrenic illness causes its patients are not to be underestimated. It takes a long time for her to recover fully, although during this time it may also be possible for her to put in a lot of effort besides her therapy, and enjoy good times with others who she knows from the hospital, for example, including as described with companions on the ward.

Countering unhappiness

Schizophrenia seems to start with the unhappiness the patient experiences in her representational world; it may be this that affects her brain, causing brain dysfunction. Dysfunction in her brain may be considered in its turn to produce further symptoms such as very disturbed language output and behaviour. Encouraging the patient to articulate her concerns as she feels these, saying exactly the meaning she wants to express, over time produces a picture her Psychoanalyst is trained to make sense of. Sometimes she may astonish herself after doing this. It may actually happen that she did not realise she felt this, or that this is the truth of her situation after all. The process of psychotherapy's efficacy has been known for a long time, but its relevance to schizophrenic illness is only now becoming better understood. Schizophrenic symptoms can for long periods mask the patient's self beneath them. Overcoming them is hard work, and time has to be allowed for this. If a patient makes no progress or very little progress over time, then the treatment may not be successful if continued; but sometimes, with warmth and encouragement, the illness may be penetrated. The full results may not be seen for at least a decade following treatment. But the early stages of breaking down the grip the illness has on the patient's mind are seminal in her life's chances. Her illness may have arisen from a very unpleasant or cruel interaction between a feature of her representational world's environment during her development and an unconscious thought, that she had been completely unaware of, that had lain hidden in her mind for most of her adult life. Only the hard work that she puts in with her Psychoanalyst, and all of his skills and dedication to her, has the chance of letting her discover her own truths about herself; these could have been inhibiting her from functioning normally, preventing her from experiencing happily or productively the perfectly basic processes of life. It is very sad for her to be saddled with these difficulties; but this treatment has the potential to let her overcome them if she works consistently at it herself.

Steady continuity

Steady continuity in the long term for the schizophrenic or schizoaffective patient in her hospital provision and therapy is key to eroding the illness' effects on her. Her circumstances will change, and she will move into different environments; but the core process of stopping to think; reflecting; observing; concluding; and changing, which she has learnt on her ward and with her Psychoanalyst, she will be fully able to adopt for herself without supervision right through the rest of her life. Psychoanalytic psychotherapy has been described as "the gift that goes on giving". This is a true description. The numerical effect sizes of psychoanalytic psychotherapy as statistics are multiples of times greater than for other types of psychological therapy, over a wide range of mental health disorders. One of the main reasons for this is exactly this: the benefits continue for years afterwards, because the patient becomes her own therapist, her own best friend. She may benefit from further help, but the illness, including when this is schizophrenia, has ceased to dominate her thinking; the patient has been educated or trained in how to recognise its offending habits, its tendencies to hurt her in her mind, so the patient can then compensate for this or put up with it for the time being, knowing that "that's all this experience is" – it's how her mind works. The time and care spent by her Psychoanalyst educating her as to this really does have a permanent effect on the patient who has listened to him. Dr Robbins selected his patients partly for their intelligence and willingness to work hard. But in addition to this, a transference that enables trust to develop between the Psychoanalyst and his patient over the long term, where both independently find reward as the patient starts to "thaw" out of her condition, is perhaps the best indication of possible success in the future.

References

Argyle, M (1987). *The Psychology of Happiness*, 2nd Edn. Hove: Routledge.

Huppert, F; Baylis, N; Keverne, B (2005). *The Science of Well-Being*. Oxford: Oxford University Press.

Robbins, M (1993). Experiences of Schizophrenia: An Integration of the Personal, Scientific and Therapeutic. New York: Guilford Press.

Glossary

Affect: emotion.

Analysand: the patient.

Auto-erotism: where the patient finds themselves sexually attractive.

Cathexis: emotional investment in a person or a thing.

Countertransference: feelings a Psychoanalyst may experience for their patient.

Defence mechanism: a measure that the mind's ego adopts to protect itself when it feels under threat from aspects of other people. There are many examples, such as splitting, projection, projective identification, repression, intellectualization, and displacement.

Depressive position: a state of mind where another person is regarded in the round, with both good and bad attributes, and where the patient feels guilty and wishes to make reparations to the other for any hurt they may have caused to them.

Differentiation: becoming a unique, characterized individual different from others.

Ego: the individual, personal self.

Individuation: becoming an integrated and unique individual.

Internalization: taking in, by adoption, into the patient's self an entity such as a feeling, an idea, or another person's identity as an internal object.

Internal object: a person whom the patient has internalized, or metaphorically taken into themselves, and who exists psychologically within the patient and can influence them during the person's absence from the patient.

Introjection: taking into oneself through internalization.

Libido: the patient's appetitive energy and interest.

"Links":   Wilfred Bion's "Links" of Love, Hate, and Knowledge are bonds, with other people, that he saw schizophrenic patients destroying as part of their illness. These bonds are formed by healthy people with others and sustain them in their normal, everyday relationships with others during life. Love, Hate, and Knowledge summarise as broad categories of the characteristics of these bonds.

Mentalising: imaginatively perceiving and interpreting behaviour of oneself and others as conjoined with intentional mental states, i.e. "holding mind in mind".

Narcissism: a mental state where the patient's mental energy and investment are directed inwards.

Object: a person other than the patient to whom the patient relates.

Object relationship: the patient's relationship with another object (another person) or with an internal object within her ego.

Oedipus conflict: an early process in an infant's life when relations with the father as well as with the mother become stabilized, with some tension, into the adult pattern.

Oral-Sadistic: an aggressive early infantile stage of development.

Paranoid: a state of mind, or a patient experiencing it, where the patient is anxious about being attacked; and which may initiate an unjustified attack on a feared person in deluded self-defence.

Paranoid-schizoid position: a state of mind where the patient regards another person as all good or all bad, as extremes of perceptual experience which bear no relation to each other. The patient's mind has become split into different parts as a defence mechanism which prevents the patient from functioning as a capable, strong individual. In this state, the patient commonly suffers from considerable paranoid anxiety.

Phantasy: freely roaming unconscious mental activity.

PPCC model: the shapes of a schizoaffective patient's mind as it recovers into mental health, as illustrated by the PPCC Theory.

PPCC Theory: the changes a schizoaffective patient's mind undergoes as it recovers into health through psychoanalytic psychotherapy may be illustrated accurately, and conceptually visualized, as geometric shapes.

The PPCC/PPCC construct: the pentapointed PPCC shape.

Projection: an emotional impulse is extended towards an object.

Projective identification: a defence mechanism common in schizophrenic patients where bad feelings in the patient are unconsciously evacuated out of themselves and into another person. This may lead to the patient disowning the feelings and the other person experiencing the feelings rather than the patient. The patient may attribute part of the self to an object.

Representation: the representative presence of the self or another object in the ego.

Splitting: a defence mechanism where the patient's mind becomes separated into different parts which may be contradictory towards each other, e.g. good and bad perceptions of another person.

Symbiotic phase: a very early phase of development in which a baby and its mother are highly interdependent.

Teleological: the capacity only to interpret phenomena or events in terms of their purpose rather than possible causes.

Therapeutic alliance: the working relationship between the Psychoanalyst and the patient.

Thing-cathexis: emotional investment in a thing.

Transference: the personal feelings that the patient may develop for the Psychoanalyst. The transference may be positive (agreeable) or negative (antagonistic).

Word-cathexis: emotional investment in a word.

Index

Note: **Bold** page numbers refer to tables; *italic* page numbers refer to figures.

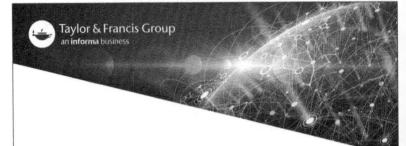

For Product Safety Concerns and Information please contact our EU
representative GPSR@taylorandfrancis.com Taylor & Francis Verlag GmbH,
Kaufingerstraße 24, 80331 München, Germany

Printed and bound by CPI Group (UK) Ltd, Croydon, CR0 4YY
08/06/2025
01897000-0005